I0425764

PSYCHEDELICS
FOR BEGINNERS

Treat PTSD, Drug Addiction, Depression, and Expand Your Mind - Using Ayahuasca, Magic Mushrooms, DMT, MDMA, LSD, and more

By: Jacob Sloan

© Copyright 2019 - All rights reserved.

The content contained within this book may not be reproduced, duplicated or transmitted without direct written permission from the author or the publisher.

Under no circumstances will any blame or legal responsibility be held against the publisher, or author, for any damages, reparation, or monetary loss due to the information contained within this book. Either directly or indirectly.

Legal Notice:

This book is copyright protected. This book is only for personal use. You cannot amend, distribute, sell, use, quote or paraphrase any part, or the content within this book, without the consent of the author or publisher.

Disclaimer Notice:

Please note the information contained within this document is for educational and entertainment purposes only. All effort has been executed to present accurate, up to date, and reliable, complete information. No warranties of any kind are declared or implied. Readers acknowledge that the author is not engaging in the rendering of legal, financial, medical or professional advice. The content within this book has been derived from various sources. Please consult a licensed professional before attempting any techniques outlined in this book.

By reading this document, the reader agrees that under no circumstances is the author responsible for any losses, direct or indirect, which are incurred as a result of the use of information contained within this document, including, but not limited to, — errors, omissions, or inaccuracies.

Table of Contents

Introduction

There has always been and will most likely always be great controversy over drug use. Even when some drugs are shown to benefit individuals, they are still criticized for being used. There are also always going to be concerns over the safety and effectiveness of drugs that are available and being tested. Some drugs are known to pose serious risks to those who use them but they are still used, for example, someone who is addicted to heroin, someone who drinks too much, or an individual suffering from depression and just looking for an escape. There are also always going to be companies that provide drugs they know can have serious side effects on those who use them; prescription painkillers and stimulants are some of the most prescribed drugs in the United States and often come with serious side effects when taking them.

In the early 1950s there were groundbreaking drugs that were shown to be highly effective with little negative side effects when used. They were viewed as "miracle drugs" and it was believed they would change the course of medical treatment in profound ways.

From the 1950s to the 1960's, psychedelic drugs were plentiful and many looked at them as a privilege to experience the mind-altering clarity it offered, especially the younger generation. Young adults looked at them as a rite of passage, entering the depths of their own minds in a way that many older adults would never be able to comprehend. But, just as quickly as they gained popularity, these drugs started to take on a darker identity. They were not intended to be used recreationally, in fact, a look into history shows how psychedelics had been used for thousands of years because of their unique healing properties.

Nowadays, you will find people who sit on both sides of the fence - those who think these types of drugs can work miracles and deserve to be used freely by those who choose to use them, for whatever purposes they feel the need to use them for. On the other side, individuals look at these drugs as purely dangerous and damaging, and that they should be kept away from public use no matter what the benefits may be from using them. They believe that not only is the person using them in danger but all individuals who come in contact with that person. What side of the fence are you on?

Today, there is a new wave of scientists looking at the effects of psychedelics to help treat a wide range of mental illnesses. They believe that all the negativity that surrounds these drugs can be disputed through the new advancements in technology and a greater understanding of how brain waves, chemicals, and bodily functions can be clearly affected by these psychedelics in a positive way.

This book is designed to shed light on the areas of psychedelic drugs that have been greatly overshadowed with false information and misunderstandings. Through this book you will understand how these drugs were discovered, created, first believed to change the way patients were treated for a number of medical conditions, and how quickly they were pushed aside.

This book will cover some of the most common psychedelic drugs like:

- Psilocybin

- Peyote

- LSD

- MDMA

- and many others.

Both synthetic and organic drugs will be discussed, and you will see how many organic psychedelics have a long history that is tied to traditions still used today. You will learn what these drugs were initially meant to treat, what type of experience they provide individuals, their potential for medical use and the success some have had in treating rare medical conditions.

Whether you lean to one side or the other, you are about to discover the good, the bad, and the life-changing mystery behind psychedelics.

Chapter 1:

Not All Drugs Are the Same

Before we dive into the world of psychedelic drugs, one thing must be addressed and discussed first. With the whole world and more specifically the United States all dealing with their own types of drug epidemics, there is no wonder why there is much apprehension in talking about further studying the effects and benefits of certain categories of drugs, like psychedelics. What there is much misunderstanding about, is the difference between certain drugs. Drugs tend to fall under four main categories: stimulants, depressants, opiates, and hallucinogens. These also come with subcategories and some would say there are more categories that can further separate the different drugs but these are typically the four main categories. Drugs can also fall into more than one category but each category affects individuals in different ways and this must be understood in order to have a more open mind about drugs that have a negative reputation but are actually quite beneficial.

Stimulants

Central nervous system stimulants help stimulate brain activity. They can increase both the cognitive processing system as well as the central nervous system. Stimulants are supposed to increase levels of serotonin, dopamine, and norephedrine. Some stimulants can also increase the levels of leptin, which is responsible for monitoring appetite. When levels of norephedrine and dopamine are increased, this triggers blood pressure, blood glucose, blood vessel constriction, and causes the heart rate to increase.

Stimulants are commonly used to help treat a number of mental disorders like:

- Attention Deficit Disorder (ADD)

- Lethargy

- Obesity

- Narcolepsy

- Apnea

- Postural Orthostatic Tachycardia Syndrome

They often cause individuals to feel:

- More energetic

- More alert

- More focused

- More excited

- More talkative

- More active

The most common stimulants include:

- Caffeine

- Amphetamine (Dyanavel)

- Dextroamphetamine (Adderall)

- Cocaine

Stimulants are favored by college students as they can help them stay up for longer periods of time and help them focus.

When taken in high doses, the result can be fatal. Additionally, these types of drugs are considered addictive and have serious withdrawal symptoms. Addictions can develop after just a few uses of these. There can also be a tolerance that is developed when taking these drugs, resulting in individuals having to take more to feel the effects which can result in overdosing and death.

Stimulants may also cause paranoia or psychosis.

Depressants

Depressants affect the central nervous system. They increase gamma-aminobutyric acid neurotransmitters which are responsible for sending signals and messages to cells in the body. This causes individuals to become more relaxed as the body slows down on depressants due to slowing of neurological functions.

Depressants or sedatives are used to help treat:

- Anxiety

- Sleep disorders

- Social phobia

- Panic disorders

- Obsessive-Compulsive Disorder

- Depression

- Seizures

They were considered harmless and effective forms of treatment in the early 90s but it was discovered that these drugs could easily be abused and often lead to overdosing. While they have been found to be an effective form of treatment for short-term success, because of the high risk of addiction they are not considered an option to help with long-term treatment (Cherry, 2019).

Depressants often cause individuals to feel:

- More relaxed

- More mellow

- Calmer

- Drowsy

The most common depressants include alcohol, benzodiazepines, and barbiturates.

These drugs can also cause an increase in aggression, anxiety, and can cause sleep disturbances.

Opioids/Opiates

Opiates and opioids depress the central nervous system and are obtained from poppy plants or semi-synthetic alkaloids. They are designed to adhere to certain brain receptors to trigger an effect that is similar to the one the body naturally performs when certain chemicals are released. Opiates directly affect pain signals sent to areas of the body because they block receptors from the brain, spine, and the rest of the body from sending these pain signals. These are the leading drugs involved in the drug epidemic in the United States and are causing more concern around the world.

Opioids and opiates are commonly prescribed to help with:

- Pain management

- Injury related pain

- Back pain

- Dental pai

Opioids and opiates often cause individuals to feel:

- A sudden rush of pleasure

- Feelings of being in a dream-like state

- Tiredness

Some of the most common opioids and opiates include:

- Heroin

- Oxycodone

- Codeine

- Morphine

- Prescription painkillers

Often, addiction and tolerance can occur even when someone is prescribed the drugs. When one builds up a strong enough tolerance they run a greater risk of overdosing. Many who are legally prescribed painkillers turn to more dangerous street drugs like heroin because it is either cheaper or because they can no longer get their prescription painkillers.

Hallucinogens

Hallucinogens are also known as psychedelics. These drugs often cause visual disturbance, an altered sense of reality, and out of body experiences. Hallucinogens are alkaloids because of their nitrogen compounds and are similar to the chemical structures of neurotransmitters in the brain. These types of drugs are often divided into two sub-categories: classic hallucinogens (like LSD) and dissociative drugs (like PCP).

Classic hallucinogens: These hallucinogens are typically ones that give you more vivid and distorted hallucinations. One tends to lose their sense of time and reality. LSD, Peyote, and Psilocybin are the most well-known types of classic hallucinogens.

Dissociative drugs: These hallucinogens make one feel more detached. This detachment can either be with reality or oneself or sometimes both. PCP and Ketamine are examples of dissociative drugs.

Hallucinogens often cause individuals to:

- Feel detached

- Have unusual mood swings

- Have visual distortions

- Experience a skewed perception of reality

- Feel spiritual enlightenment

- Hallucinate

- Have an altered perception of time and space

Hallucinogens can include both synthetic/man-made drugs as well as organic/from plants and nature. Common hallucinogens include:

- LSD

- MDMA (ecstasy)

- Peyote

- Psilocybin

- PCP

These types of drugs seem to carry little to known signs of addiction but individuals can become tolerant. Under the Controlled Substance Act most of these types of drugs are listed as Schedule I drugs meaning they are considered highly dangerous, unsafe, and have no medical use.

Controlled Substance Act

The Controlled Substance Act was enforced in 1970. It was created just a few years after the discovery of LSD, and was said to have been created to help regulate drugs for the safety of the general public. The act establishes how drugs can be manufactured, distributed, and used by companies, researchers, and the public. The laws established under this act were supposed to help limit access to what were considered controlled substances and would therefore reduce the risk of these substances being misused or abused.

Drugs are classified as either narcotics, depressants, anabolic steroids, stimulants, or hallucinogens according to the Controlled Substance Act. The Act categorizes substances into 5 schedules and where the drug is placed depends on:

1. How or if it can be medically used

2. How safe they are in terms of how easily people could

become dependent

3. How likely or easy it is to abuse the drug?

Schedule I Controlled Substances:

Drugs classified in the Schedule I Controlled Substance category are believed:

1. To have no medical use

2. To be safe

3. Have a high potential for abuse

The classification of "no medical use" is based off of what the federal government has approved for medical use opt treatment. This can include that the drug would still have no importance or benefit to the medical community if administered in a controlled environment or even if administered under professional supervision.

Drugs classified as Schedule I include:

- Heroin

- LSD

- Marijuana

- MDMA

- Peyote

- Psilocybin

Schedule II Controlled Substances:

Drugs classified in the Schedule II Controlled Substance category are believed:

1. To have little medical use

2. To result in a serious risk of dependency

3. To have a high potential for abuse.

The drugs in this Schedule are believed to have some medical use but must follow specific restrictions as they have a high dependency and abuse rate.

Drugs classified as Schedule II include:

- Cocaine

- Morphine

- Methadone

- Phencyclidine PCP

- Methamphetamine

Schedule III Controlled Substances:

Drugs classified in the Schedule III Controlled Substance category are believed:

1. To have a medical use

2. To have a moderate or low risk of dependency

3. To have a low risk of abuse

Drugs listed in the schedule III category are often viewed as fairly safe. They are currently used and regularly prescribed for medical purposes. Some can even be easily purchased without a prescription.

Drugs classified as Schedule III include:

- Codeine

- Tylenol

- Barbiturates

- Anabolic Steroids

Schedule IV Controlled Substances:

Drugs classified in the Schedule IV Controlled Substance category are believed:

1. To have a medical use

2. To be relatively safe with little risk of dependency

3. To have a relatively low potential for abuse

Drugs in the Schedule IV category have been proven to provide value in the medical field. They are currently used as a form of treatment. These drugs possess little to no possibility for abuse or dependency.

Drugs classified as Schedule IV include:

- Equanil

- Darvon

- Valium

- Xanax

Schedule V Controlled Substances:

Drugs classified in the Schedule V Controlled Substance category are believed:

1. To have a medical use.

2. Are safe with little to no risk of dependency

3. To have little to no potential for abuse

Drugs in the Schedule V category are viewed as the safest drugs to use. They are used regularly to treat a variety of common illnesses and are found in many homes. There is little concern that drugs in the Schedule V category will result in dependence or abuse.

Drugs classified as Schedule V include:

- Cough medicines

Research Requirements

Drugs must pass through a process in order for them to not only be distributed and manufactured in the United States, but to also be researched and tested. The first step of the process is typically to submit a proposal that will prove the drug is safe and can be effective if used. The proposal must include a plan that provides a detailed description of the type of research to be conducted and how it will be conducted. The research and process must also be proven safe and the benefits must outweigh the negative effects or risks.

Once approved, there are five to ten additional steps one must take in order to get a drug approved by the FDA. Schedule I drugs are especially difficult to obtain approval for.

Things to Keep in Mind

1. By understanding the types of drugs, how they affect people, their side effects, and how they are categorized by the Federal Government you may begin to see a few flaws in the system. These categories were initially developed in the 1970s and few amendments have been made due to the fact that Congress has full control of the rescheduling of drugs and the process can be cumbersome.

2. Many drugs were categorized as such because of political reasons even though there was either proven research that showed them to either be more beneficial and safe or proved them to be more of a danger and unsafe.

3. Psychedelics are the only category of drugs that demonstrate little to no risk of dependency, meaning it is very unlikely that individuals will become addicted to the substance.

4. Even though there was ongoing research in the past on psychedelic use, and that certain psychedelics were being used in certain situations for medical treatment, they were still classified as Schedule I substances.

5. This schedule system is not the same for many other countries. In the 1970s Europe had developed its own Scheduling system that was similar to the United States, but has since reorganized and re-classified many of the drugs.

Chapter 2:

Psychedelics for Beginners

Psychedelic drugs are often thought to be related to drugs like cocaine and heroin. However, there is very little that is similar between the two and it is comparisons like this that is often what leads to psychedelics being greatly misunderstood.

The term 'psychedelics' originated from the Greeks; some translate it to mean "soul manifesting", while others translate it to mean "mind" and "make visible" or "make the mind visible". Psychedelics have the ability to alter the cognitive and perceptive states of the mind. They are also better known as hallucinogenic or hallucinogens.

Psychedelics fall into the drug category of hallucinogens, and there are various subcategories of psychedelics. Many of these drugs have the same effects on individuals which include distinctly affecting their sensory perception, emotions, and immediate environment.

As a hallucinogen, psychedelics are also further classified under two distinct categories: Dissociatives and Deliriants, where the users will have an altered form of consciousness out of the norm and is often described as a dream-like state.

Dissociatives - These types of drugs cause a detachment to or disassociation of reality. Users tend to experience hallucinations and have out of body experiences.

Deliriants - These drugs will create confusion of the mind. Users tend to suffer from a state of delirium.

As a precaution, those wishing to experiment with psychedelics must have an understanding that each person experiences the effects of psychedelics differently. Each user can even produce different effects, even when taking the same psychedelic. Psychedelics have a way of bringing to light untouched, repressed, and unwanted memories or thoughts. Individuals who wish to take psychedelics must prepare themselves for these types of experiences.

There are three compound categories of psychedelic drugs as well; tryptamines, phenethylamines, and lysergamides.

Tryptamines: These compound structures are derived from tryptamine, which includes neurotransmitters, and serotonin. LSD, Psilocybin mushrooms and DMT are closely related to these compound structures.

Phenethylamines: These are compounds that can act as stimulants, hallucinogens, and entactogens. They can be both synthetic or organic. MDMA is the most well-known psychedelic that fall into this compound structure.

Lysergamides: These compounds are composed of tryptamine and phenethylamine structures. The most well-known psychedelic that is classified in this compound category is LSD.

Psychedelics can be dangerous because of their volatile side effects as well as their unpredictability. Many psychedelic drugs only pose a mild to moderate effect on users but some can have life-altering effects that come with serious consequences. These three categories of psychedelics have varying effects on state of mind and in the way it alters perception. As with many drugs, there are both synthetic or chemical psychedelics and natural or organic psychedelics.

Psychedelics affect the activity of neurotransmitters which they have chemical similarities with. A chemical imbalance occurs when taking a psychedelic, which is why users will experience hallucinations, an increase in sensory processing, and hyper-awareness. The 5-HT2A receptors are directly affected by some psychedelics, while the neuron structure of the brain is affected by other psychedelics (Olsen, ND).

Chemical/Synthetic Psychedelics

Synthetic psychedelics can produce and often do produce the same effects as natural psychedelics. They are man-made substances which are often better related to amphetamines than their natural counterparts. These psychedelics are known as N-bombs or N-methoxybenzyl, NBOMe (An Overview on Synthetic Hallucinogens, 2019).

When these psychedelic drugs were first researched, they were based on an attempt to understand the brain's serotonin receptors, however, they quickly became a recreational drug among the general population.

Synthetic psychedelics can have minor to severe side effects. Since these drugs affect serotonin in the brain which is responsible for regulating mood and sensory input according to the National Institute of Drug Abuse, they can have varying effects on a person. The Drug Enforcement Administration lists some of these effects as:

- Hallucinations

- Increase in heart rate

- Highly active sensory perceptions

- Loss of time

- Higher blood pressure

- Trouble sleeping

- State of relaxation

- Detachment

- Loss of appetite

- Loss of balance or coordination

- State of panic

- Paranoia

- Sweating

- Unclear thought process

These side effects present themselves within half an hour to one hour of taking the psychedelic and can last for hours. While uncommon, there can also be long-term effects from using these psychedelics. Kidney and bladder issues are rare but are the most common long-term effects as well as memory impairment.

Natural/Organic Psychedelics

Almost all psychedelics, synthetic or organic, originate from plants. The most common and most potent of these plants are fungi, which account for over 100 hallucinogenic plants. These psychedelics can be administered a number of ways and prepared even in even more ways. Some are smoked, swallowed, sniffed, infused, dried, taken fresh, or applied to the skin. Organic or natural psychedelics are extracted directly from the source. Most are taken from the seeds of various plants or resin from bark, and rare psychedelics are obtained from the poisonous venom of animals such as the Colorado River Toad.

Organic psychedelics will affect individuals in many of the same ways synthetic psychedelics affect individuals. These types of psychedelics, however, tend to produce more intense hallucinations. Carbon dating has found evidence of psychedelic use as early as 5000 years ago. Peyote and iboga are among the first psychedelic drugs discovered in written scriptures.

Chapter 3:

Misconceptions and Myths of Psychedelics

Just mentioning the word psychedelic can conjure up images of swirling colors and moving objects that should be stationary. Maybe you think of Alice in Wonderland? Crowds of people at Woodstock? Maybe you conjure up a more traumatic situation where seemingly harmless people just snap? The truth is, while psychedelics can cause individuals to see vivid colors, moving pictures, and out of character behavior, there is also a great deal that most people believe that is actually completely untrue. While some things may have been perceived as the truth at the time when psychedelics were first being used by the general public, it is these strongly held misconceptions that have been hindering the progress of finding out the benefits that psychedelics can offer to many individuals. Some of the most common misconceptions and myths that surround psychedelics are discussed below.

Misconception number one: Psychedelics put those who use them and others in danger

Many people believe that taking a psychedelic can increase the risk of injury or reckless behavior. This misconception was heightened due to the fact that most reports that were made public concerning psychedelics over-emphasized the outrageous behavior some individuals exhibited. While psychedelics do have a psychological effect on the user those who are only likely to be at risk of harming themselves or others are individuals who have serious mental or psychological disorders. User experiences can result in instability and interfere with mental clarity but this is typical and does not result in the user being more likely to harm themselves or others due to this. Since psychedelics can bring to light a number of suppressed thoughts, emotions, and memories, individuals that tend to suppress these uncomfortable thoughts can often become significantly overwhelmed by them when on a psychedelic. This is what increases the risk of negative, dangerous, or harmful behavior during the first phases of a psychedelic experience. These drugs were originally intended to be taken under the supervision of medical professionals in a calm and relaxed environment. When taken in the right setting and in the right state of mind as well as having a clear understanding of how these drugs can affect you there is no danger imposed on the users or those around the user.

Misconception number two: Psychedelics are addictive

When you attach the word 'drug' to anything that can be used recreationally there is a tendency for public opinion to sway towards a negative view. Psychedelics are more often than not considered to be addictive substances. This is a common thought of many individuals when they think of psychedelic drugs. Psychedelics, however, are not addictive. Unlike other drugs that are highly addictive, like opioids and heroin, psychedelics affect the serotonin receptors in the brain. Opioids and heroin directly affect the dopamine receptors which trigger the reward system of the brain; this is why they create intense feelings and attachment to the drugs. Psychedelics do not trigger this reward system.

This does not, however, mean they are completely harmless. Psychedelics can be easily abused or simply taken in the wrong setting. Taking a psychedelic when you are with the wrong people, in the wrong environment, or not emotionally stable can result in dangerous outcomes. If one recognizes the dangers of their environment or the people they are with prior to taking a psychedelic and avoids taking them in these situations they are less likely to have a bad experience.

Additionally, psychedelics can be abused when continuously taken in these types of settings. Individuals will often feel a "need" to take psychedelics to confront certain people or situations which results in more negative feelings towards them. It can be easy to fall into a bad trip cycle where one just wants to "escape" from their reality. This is not considered addiction as there are no withdrawal symptoms when the user goes without taking the drugs as is common when one is addicted to other types of substances.

While they do have a powerful effect on the mind, most classic psychedelics have no addictive components. They are not toxic, are considered to be safer than consuming alcohol, and many are actually the safest psychoactive substances used. LSD and magic mushrooms (psilocybin mushrooms) are also four times safer to use than tobacco products (What are Psychedelics?, ND). Using psychedelics has even been shown to lower the risk of psychological conditions.

Misconception number three: Psychedelics are only popular among the younger generations and pose no medical benefits

There is a common opinion that many psychedelic drugs, especially LSD, Ecstasy, and mushrooms, are primarily party or "club" drugs. Though these drugs are common in the club scene, that is not how they are commonly used or were intended to be used. In cultures around the world, and even in the United States, psychedelic drugs are used in spiritual ceremonies, or to obtain a deeper connection with the world around us. In the medical field, these drugs are continuously experimented with to help treat a number of serious mental and psychological disorders.

Misconception number four: Psychedelics cause individuals to have intense experiences

Every time you take a psychedelic you will experience a 'trip'. While psychedelics are widely known for the effects they have on a person, causing hallucinations, heightened sense, and greater awareness, these are not always experienced when taking a psychedelic drug. Taking a full dose of a psychedelic drug will induce these side effects, but taking much smaller doses will not produce these common 'trip' effects on the user.

Misconception number five: Psychedelics will cause holes to form in the brain

Thanks to anti-drug ads in the early 80s, many think of psychedelics and think of eggs frying in a pan. The idea that psychedelics cause holes to form in the brain would indicate that those who use psychedelic drugs all experienced some form of severe brain trauma. Long-term use of psychedelic drug use is believed to cause long-term damage to the brain. Many believe that psychedelic drugs will damage the brain the same way many other recreational drugs tend to do.

Studies, in contrast, show that psychedelics can actually reduce the possibility of mental illness developing later in life.

A case study published on PubMed compared three groups of Navajo Native Americans. The study focused on the effect peyote had on the brains of lifetime users compared to the effect alcohol had on a group of heavy drinkers and the progress of the brains of individuals in the third group who only occasionally used alcohol or peyote. The RMHI scale, neuropsychological test on memory, and attention and executive function test indicated that those in the peyote lifetime group had no decrease in neurological function throughout the study. Those in the alcohol consumption group had a significant decrease in every area of brain function (Halpern, Hudson, Pope, Sherwood, Yurgelun, 2005).

Misconception number six: The banning of psychedelics was primarily due to a concern for public safety

The Nixon campaign started their "War on Drugs" efforts in the late 1960s and early 1970s which claimed that psychedelic drugs were dangerous and that there were no facts that suggested they could produce any beneficial medical breakthroughs. Nixon would publicly attack those who encouraged the general public to use psychedelic drugs; though it was said to be for public health safety reasons, it was later revealed that the efforts of the Nixon campaign to stop psychedelic drug use was nothing more than a hidden political agenda. Its purpose was to separate and diminish the power of specific groups by painting these groups as dangerous and a burden on society.

A year before the Watergate Scandal in 1971, the Nixon campaign declared drugs as the number one enemy of the United States. A few months later in early 1972, ODALE, the Office of Drug Abuse Law Enforcement, which would later develop into what is currently known as the DEA, along with a number of other anti-drug agencies, were created to gain a handle on the drug epidemic taking over America. According to John Ehrlichman, who was appointed as Assistant for Domestic Affairs while Nixon was in office, the real war was against the anti-war left and the black population in America (Lopez, 2016) The Nixon staff found a loophole in order to break these two groups apart. The anti-war left consisted of "hippies" and it was well-known that these individuals regularly took part in recreational drug use, so the staff then associated a majority of heroin use to those in the black community. By waging a war on drugs the staff was able to take down and disrupt these communities in a way that left them with little power to influence how others would vote.

This has created serious consequences in the present where the black community has been blamed for a great deal of the drug epidemic that plagues the United States in the present day. At the time, however, the ploy worked and Nixon and his staff were able to turn the spotlight momentarily away from the corruption that was occurring in the white house. When the United States waged its war on drugs, a number of other countries followed suit.

Chapter 4:

History of Psychedelics

Psychedelics are characterized by their ability to alter perception, senses, thoughts, and feelings. How exactly did a substance that can cause such profound alteration and be reported to have life-changing effects on individuals come into use? While some may have been accidentally engineered in labs, many others grow naturally in nature and have been a part of history for hundreds of thousands of years.

The Western World's Introduction to Psychedelics

In 1918, researchers and scientists began to extract the compounds of plants at the Sandoz Laboratory. It was in this lab that scientists successfully extracted the ergotamine chemical compound from the fungus ergot. While the fungus can be deadly if consumed as is, when consumed in powder form in low doses it was believed to have healing properties. When scientists tested this theory, they found blood vessels were narrowed when the ergotamine chemical was introduced to the body. From this understanding, they believed this could help treat migraines. The chemical compound was purified and used successfully for many, years. It was from this first extracted compound that synthetic compounds were chemically engineered in laboratories, and it was from this compound that Hofman had accidentally created LSD.

The beginning of psychedelic drug research first began a few years after the discovery of LSD. When Albert Hofmann accidentally created LSD in 1938, he looked at it as a failed attempt to create a stimulant that would activate the circulatory system. Hofmann at the time was a physicist at the pharmaceutical firm, Sandon. Hofmann had not intended to create a powerful psychedelic drug but instead, was attempting to find a way to improve circulation in the body.

For this reason, he simply set his new discovery aside. Five years later he revisited the creation and had accidentally absorbed some of the substance through his skin. After experiencing the effects, Hofmann understood that this new drug could open up doors to various treatments.

Hofmann had begun to send samples of LSD as well as psilocybin (magic mushrooms), to various research centers and universities. The research conducted on these drugs gave scientists a greater understanding of the brain and its neurochemistry. With these discoveries, therapists were feeling more confident in how they could more effectively treat mental disorders.

One of the people who received these drugs for research was Timothy Leary. Timothy Leary was a psychologist at Harvard at the time, and it was 1960 when he began the Harvard Psilocybin Project. The project was created to study the effects of psilocybin, and although Leary was fired for distributing the drugs to undergraduates, he did not let this deter him from continuing his research in his efforts to encourage young adults to take LSD.

Although LSD and psilocybin were being primarily used in scientific experiments and research in the mental health community, little was known of the two mind-altering drugs but these two would begin a new revolution in the mental health profession. It was in the 1950s that brain science was starting to gain great attention, neurotransmitters were being understood more, psychotherapy was being introduced as a treatment for a number of disorders, and both LSD and psilocybin were being praised as miracle drugs (Pollan, 2018).

Over the next decade and a half, extensive testing was done with promising results. Thousands of papers were written and thousands of patients were administered LSD in addition to therapy showing how psychedelic treatment could change how depression, trauma, addiction, and terminal illnesses would be treated. Psychedelic treatments tended to show greater achievements where other drugs and therapies were ineffective. The CIA was also said to have performed their own testing on how effective these drugs could be when used for mind control.

At this point, the US was under great turbulence. Young adults were rebelling more against the Vietnam war and societal norms. In 1966, although there were obvious therapeutic benefits from taking psychedelic drugs, all research and distribution of psychedelics had been stopped and banned. Stories started to circulate about "bad" trips, erratic behavior, and even murder being caused by the drug's side effects. While some therapists and psychologists still administered LSD to their patients, they did so illegally and further psychedelic therapy was forced to be done secretively.

With psychedelics being viewed as dangerous and unstable, some therapists began to look into and incorporate different methods in order to mimic the psychedelic experience. In 1970, Stanislav Grof began using holotropic breathwork in his practices. This was a technique that required patients to control their breathing in a way where their breathing patterns could have an influence over the individual's physical, emotional, and mental state.

This also was not a new idea, holotropic breathing was

already being used in many countries as a spiritual practice to heighten one's awareness, similar to the use of psychedelics. Grof began to use this technique as a way to help patients suffering from cancer, psychiatric illness, and addiction. Through this practice, the patient is able to begin the process of healing from within, where the patient accesses important memories on their own that will lead them to feel empowered and bring about enlightenment. Each patient is different, and it is the patient who determines what memories to focus on. The whole process can take three or more hours.

The idea around holotropic breathwork is that one can obtain an altered state of mind by rapidly increasing and slowing the breath. This can lead to seeing things more clearly in the present moment, colors being more vivid, increase in self-awareness, and experiencing the conscious mind on a deeper level. The benefits and risks are very similar to the ones with psychedelic drugs. When you are in a trusting environment, the experience can be highly beneficial. A number of patients begin a deeper healing process after they have gone through a holotropic breathwork session. But, just like with psychedelic drugs, this technique can be harmful to those in a highly distressed state of mind and can lead to psychosis. Because of some of the negative side effects, this isn't something that should be done alone. Instead, at least two people should perform the technique, one being the sitter and the other being the breather. The sitter is purely there to ensure the breather does not enter a dangerous state of panic or has negative effects from changing their breathing pattern.

Unfortunately, not much research has been done on this practice as a viable method to help treat illnesses. It is believed that this practice, along with additional therapy, can be beneficial. While Grof was trying to implement this holotropic breathwork into his practices, another scientist was going in a different direction. Though psychedelics had been banned in the US, that did not stop scientists or chemists in other countries from experimenting with psychedelics.

In 1976, Alexander Shulgin synthesized MDMA, more commonly known as Molly. He first tested the new drug out on himself and had a life-changing experience that was nothing but positive. Shulgin eagerly sent a sample to Leo Zeff, a therapist practicing in San Francisco at the time. Despite the United States' ban on psychedelic drugs, Zeff sent samples of MDMA to other therapists, and in the 1970s, hundreds of thousands of patients were given MDMA because of its therapeutic effects. But, once again, MDMA made its way into the hands of the general public and new horror stories began to circulate of young adults become severely overheated in clubs and rumors of the drug surely rotting their brains.

MDMA, like all other psychedelics, was classified as a Schedule I drug and was banned in the US. Up until the early 2000s psychedelic testing, research and treatment had been kept quiet. Scientists and researchers would have to battle through a number of obstacles to get any kind of support for psychedelic drug testing. But, from 2006 to the present day more and more positive feedback has been circulating psychedelic drug use and is beginning to be viewed once again as a highly effective way to treat a number of disorders.

Names to Know

While you will be introduced to a vast number of important researchers and scientists who developed and lead the way in the medical use of psychedelics, there are still a number of specific people who are worth mentioning, some of whom were mentioned briefly. These are the people who experimented with psychedelics and discovered and educated the world about the benefits and truth about dealing with psychedelic drugs.

Albert Hofmann

Hofmann is credited as being the "father" of psychedelic drugs. He accidentally created LSD in the Sandoz Laboratories. After realizing the effects of what he had created he went on to learn and experiment with other organic psychedelics such as psilocybin, *rivea corymbosa* (soliloquio), and peyote. He was able to receive samples of new psychedelic research in his lab and was able to synthesize a number of hallucinogenic compounds. He was a leading advocate for the use of psychedelic drugs to be used in psychiatric treatment. He also wrote a number of books including:

- *LSD, My Problem Child*

- *Plants of the Gods*

- *Insight, outlook*

- *Hofmann's Elixir: LSD and the New Eleusis*

Hofmann died in 2008 at the age of 102.

Timothy Leary

Timothy Leary is probably the most well-known names in connection with psychedelic drugs. He was a psychologist and dedicated his work to develop a new model of how patient and psychotherapist should make a connection as well as creating advanced techniques to utilize in group therapy sessions. He was a lecturer at the time when he was introduced to psychedelics at Harvard University. He and Richard Alpert (now known as Ram Dass), founded the Harvard Psilocybin Project where they extensively researched the philosophical and cultural effects of psychedelic drugs. Leary adamantly encouraged the use of psychedelic drugs among the younger generation. When it was discovered he was sharing the psychedelic drugs he obtained for research purposes with the undergraduate students at Harvard he was quickly dismissed, along with Richard Alpert. Leary moved to New York where a hedonistic community formed around his research on LSD. From his research, he would devise the "set and setting" guidelines, explaining how one could create an environment that would help individuals have an enlightening and safe experience. He soon began traveling and lecturing on the topic of psychedelic drugs from which the slogan "Turn on, tune in, drop out" came about. Leary's lectures gained much attention, especially that of President Nixon who did not appreciate Leary's constant encouragement of the younger generation to take psychedelics.

Leary would be arrested a number of times for possession between 1965 and 1970. He was placed in jail in 1970 which resulted in a well-planned out escape and he was forced to flee to Algeria. He was captured in Afghanistan and returned to the United States where he was sent back to prison for three years. After his release, he began to lecture again but was unable to gain the popularity he had previously. He spent the rest of his days mostly writing various literature and memoirs, and also dabbled in computer software design. He eventually died in 1996 after a long battle with prostate cancer.

Terence McKenna

Terence McKenna was born in 1946 and is known as a philosopher, ethnobotanist (someone who studies plant lore) and lecturer, and for being a powerful figure who helped lead the psychedelic movement in the 1960s. He was in support of psychedelic drugs being used to help one form a better connection with nature and to bring about more harmony. He not only was interested in psychedelics but also how they were used culturally around the world throughout history. He encouraged more use of organic psychedelics as opposed to synthetic psychedelics as organic psychedelics bring you closer to nature.

He used art, literature, music, and other visuals to help translate his psychedelic experience to others. Some of the books Terence McKenna wrote include:

- *The Invisible Landscape*

- *Food of the Gods*

- *The Archaic Revival*

- *Psilocybin: Magic Mushrooms*

- *True Hallucinations*

Stan Grof

Stan Grof, born in 1931 in Czechoslovakia, extensively studied the effects of LSD and the impact it could have on a person's psyche. When LSD was made illegal in the 60s, he sought out alternative ways one could have the same transformative experience as they would when taking a psychedelic. Grof theorized that one could alter their own state of mind without relying on external substances. He began utilizing what he called holotropic breathwork, which was a breathing technique that could alter the state of mind of individuals similar to how LSD or MDMA could. While he did not outwardly oppose psychedelic use or their benefits he did prove that it was possible to have similar experiences which could be just as beneficial as psychedelic drugs.

Grof became a faculty member at the California Institute of Integral Studies in the Department of Philosophy, Cosmology, and Consciousness. He has also written over a hundred scientific articles and has published a number of books covering the topic of consciousness, psychology, and transformation. Some of the books Stan Grof wrote include:

- *Holotropic Breathwork*

- *The Cosmic Game: Exploration of the Frontiers of Human Consciousness*

- *When the Impossible Happens*

- *Realms of the Human Unconscious*

- *LSD Psychotherapy*

Christina Grof

Christina Grof, worked closely with her husband Stan Grof to spread awareness of the benefits of holotropic breathwork. She was a well-known author and teacher, giving lectures and running workshops around the world. She taught writing, art, and hatha yoga. Like her husband, Christina Grof wrote a number of books which include:

- *The Thirst for Wholeness: Attachment, Addiction, and the Spiritual Path*

- *The Eggshell Landing*

- *The Stormy Search for Self*

- *Holotropic Breathwork: A New Approach to Self-Exploration and Therapy*

- *Spiritual Emergency: When Personal Transformation Becomes a Crisis*

In 2014, Christina Grof died of pneumonia.

Rick Doblin

In 1982, Rick Doblin was attending an off-campus course lead by Stan and Christina Grof, where he was first introduced to MDMA and the psychedelic community. It was there that he would find himself in a number of discussions that focused on how psychedelics could be brought back for medicinal purposes. Eventually, in 1986, Rick Doblin would found the Multidisciplinary Association of Psychedelics Substances (MAPS). This organization would lead the way in spreading a positive understanding of psychedelic drugs. It was set up as a non-profit organization that would raise funds to fuel the research that would show the advantages psychedelic drugs could provide to the medical community.

Unlike much of the research being done at the time, MAPS was not going against the system. Psychedelics were illegal at the time MAPS was first created and it was almost impossible to gain approval for any type of medical testing, trials, or research. Rick Doblin used his political upbringing to guide MAPS to become a leading resource for much of the information that was generated on the safety and effectiveness of psychedelic drugs. In the beginning years, he focused on gathering a number of peer reviews that would help support their mission. Once they had what he believed was enough material to back up their hypothesis on specific psychedelics, they began the long process to gain approval for research and trials. MAPS worked closely with government agencies instead of opposing them, which allowed the organization to clearly understand the guidelines and procedures to gain access to psychedelic drugs. All this effort would eventually pay off and MAPS would be granted permission to begin research on a number of psychedelic drugs. It is also through their efforts that a few of these drugs had been approved for medicinal use or are close to gaining FDA approval.

Amanda Feilding

Amanda Feilding founded *The Foundation to Further Consciousness* in 1996, which would later become The Beckley Foundation. Feilding first understood the benefits of psychedelic drugs when she was introduced to them in the 1960s. After her first experience, she began researching and learning about the potential that psychedelics offered to treat and cure various illness. She developed The Beckley

Foundation in order to use up to date technology like brain imaging software, that would show the direct effect psychedelics had on the function and structure of the brain. It was her mission to gather data to show how researchers and scientists could better understand and test the effectiveness of psychedelic drugs in the medical field.

Through her efforts, she was able to gain support, attention, and priceless evidence that proved the previously held opinion on psychedelics, that being they had no medical use and were highly dangerous, was inaccurate. Through the foundation, she was able to not only collect data but also publish countless reports, books, papers, and more that were made accessible to the general public so they too could realize the misconception they held about psychedelic drugs. Her research was able to help other organizations and groups gather the data they needed to obtain approval for psychedelic testing. It is also this data that is helping change the laws and policies that restrict the testing and research done on psychedelic drugs.

Psychedelics in Other Cultures and Societies

Psilocybin, a little brown mushroom, was used by indigenous people who made a home of Central America and parts of Mexico. They used it in rituals and sacraments, but when the Roman Catholic Church became aware of the rituals it was used in, they quickly suppressed it and for years it was hidden and rarely spoken of until 1955.

R. Gordon Wasson was one of the first individuals from the Western world to bring back and publicly share his experience with magic mushrooms a few years after his return from the small town of Huautla de Jimenez. Many tribes, cultures, and spiritual groups use psychedelics on a regular basis. These drugs aren't used for recreational use but instead are deeply rooted in tradition. While western society had started to look at the medicinal benefits these drugs could provide, many cultures had already used and experienced these benefits without having to do years of research or testing. It is easier to pinpoint the beginning of synthetic psychedelic drugs as data, reports, and concrete evidence gives a clear and precise timeline for when these drugs were created. But cave drawing, carbonate fossils, and written documents can trace organic psychedelic drug use back for thousands of years.

Babongo Tribe

Over a thousand years ago, the Babongo Tribe first discovered the effects of the Iboga Plant. This plant primarily grows along the western coast of Central Africa near Gabon. The plant, resembling a shrub, is distinguishable by its white or pink flowers and produces an orange fruit that lacks flavor. Though the plant adds little visual appeal or nutritional benefits, the Babongo tribe has labeled it as one of their sacred shrubs. Their religion, Bwiti, was formed around the powerful effects the root bark of this shrub had on them. Spiritual growth and community strength were gained from the rituals that involved this bark, which was typically ground into a fine powder or shaved into chips. Ceremonies were performed where all members of the tribe, young and old, would either partake in or watch for what the bark would reveal to them. Shamans were in charge of translating what the visuals meant from those experiencing them to the rest of the tribe. Most often these ceremonies or rituals could last up to 48 hours, as this is how long the effects of the Iboga would tend to last. Drum-filled music, chants, and clapping would fill the air as the ceremony proceeded.

The Bwiti religion used Iboga as a sacrament during weekly ceremonies. These ceremonies began on Saturday night, members dressed in colorful costumes, dances are performed, and music is played throughout the night and into the early morning of Sunday. Iboga is passed around to the members to increase the level of joy and bring in a deeper connection within the community.

When a new member wishes to join the Bwiti community, they go through a type of initiation process where they must take a higher dose of Iboga. These are similar to ceremonies that are performed to help assist another member that is going through a difficult time or when a member reaches a certain age. Ceremonies of this nature will often last for three days. Community members give extra attention to those taking the ibogaine, the psychedelic substance from the iboga plant, in these ceremonies as the high dose will often cause the individual to have an intense experience during the process. Once these ceremonies are completed, the participants will feel a sense of clarity and a high level of spirituality. The participants share their experience with the community so the whole tribe can reflect and find lessons to apply to their daily lives from the experience of others.

Ibogaine was said to be first introduced into the Western world when a young man, Howard Lotsof, publicly shared his experience with the plant which he credited to helping him beat his heroin addiction.

Ayahuasca Ceremonies

The Mestizo population and indigenous people in the Amazon region in South America take part in what can be viewed as a purging ceremony. A shaman begins the ceremony by singing traditional songs dedicated to Mother Earth as individuals consume a mixture of ayahuasca cine, chacruna leaves, jimson weed and jungle tobacco that has been boiled for 12 hours. The mixture is blessed before the ceremony begins to invite Mother Earth into the bodies of those who consume it. The ceremony is not as lively as that of the Babongo tribe, as this ceremony focuses on purging the body both figuratively and literally. Participants go through long periods of vomiting and have uncontrollable bowel movements while also experiencing vivid hallucinations. The six-hour-long ordeal is said to be one that not only physically cleanses the body but cleanses the mind and brings on transformation healing.

Shipibo Tradition

The Shipibo tribe are the natives of Peru who inhabit the Amazonian rainforest. This tribe has upheld traditions for centuries that incorporate the ayahuasca brew, a strong organic psychedelic that combines the components of two plants: the Banisteriopsis caapi and P. viridis. Ceremonies that include the ayahuasca brew are highly celebrated and much preparation goes into them. A shaman, or curanderos as titled by the Shipibo, is called upon to oversee the ceremony because the knowledge they obtained was directly from the plants. This knowledge allowed the shaman to understand and translate each individual experience on a much deeper and spiritual level.

Prior to the ceremony, participants follow a strict diet that cuts out sugar, oil, and salt. The shaman is responsible for preparing the ayahuasca brew and properly blessing it before it is consumed by the participants. Ceremonies would often begin in the evening with a welcoming of the ayahuasca spirit. The shaman will also consume the ayahuasca and use tobacco smoke to encourage positive energy to flow among the group. Songs are sung to throughout the ceremony to help ease the long journey for participants.

Other healing ceremonies would also be performed by the tribe. In these ceremonies, participants would not drink the ayahuasca brew, only the shaman would. This is because the shaman is the one who possesses the healing powers but the ayahuasca brew is what assists him.

Aztecs, Mexican Indians, and Native Americans

For over 5000 years, Mescalito has been a part of many tribes local to Northeastern Mexico and the southern border of Texas. Communal ceremonies that are both spiritual and cultural and lead by a shaman, take place regularly. It is in these ceremonies that groups of individuals are guided through an experience involving Mescalito, or what is better known as Peyote. This psychedelic is obtained from a small cactus plant that is often hidden under the ground. Ceremonies that involve Peyote can last up to 12 hours and participants tend to undergo wild hallucinations that cause the user to lose track of time and space. It is an emotional experience where participants will often confront some of their deepest fears. Though it can be a frightening experience, it is also an enlightening one where the participant seems to fully embrace and understand themselves, forming a deeper connection to the world around them, especially with nature. While the possession of Peyote is strictly banned in America, there are some instances where Peyote can be used for religious ceremonies in a select number of states.

Polynesian and Pacific Islanders

For those residing on the Pacific Island, in Hawaii, Fiji, or Vanuatu, Yaqona is simply a part of everyday life. Better known as Kava, the roots are pounded to extract a milky substance which is then consumed. Kava is taken socially and for sacred purposes, especially for entering a state of deep meditation. The effects of this plant are mild where the user remains alert and able to focus but more with a calm, still mind. This is one of the only substances that falls into the psychedelic category that is legal to consume in the United States, primarily because of its more subdued and non-disturbing effects on the mind. When one consumes Kava with the right mindset they can experience a profound enlightening experience as they would with one of the other psychedelics but without the intense mind alterations and hallucinations.

Mazatec

Before Psilocybin mushrooms became mainstream in America, this little fungus was a sacred part of the Mazatec tradition. The mushroom was used for medicinal treatment, and for healing rituals that focus on the physical, mental, and ethical values of the individual. Mazatec people would participate in communal ceremonies where a shaman would serve as a mediator. The psilocybin mushroom would be prepared by going through an incense cloud bath, then participants would consume two of the mushrooms. Taking two at a time was said to bring a connection to the male and female aspects of the universe and nature.

Ancient Indian Practices

The Hindu and Zoroastrian traditions are filled with mentions of a powerful mixture that was of great importance in religious ceremonies. The drink was known as soma and was said to provide individuals with a vivid experience that increased awareness. There have been reports of mythical settings being explored that have brought on feelings of euphoria and immortality. It was never made clear if the beverage really existed or if it was just a made up component in a fascinating tale but the stories caught the attention of R. Gordon Wasson, who is credited for introducing the Western world to psilocybin. Wasson believed Soma must have come from a psychedelic mushroom, based off of scriptures that described the plant, but others disagreed and said that it had to come from a flowering plant and not a fungus, with stems that would produce the juice for the soma mixture.

Others believe soma was not so mystifying as they believed the plant described was the common cannabis plant. The stimulant qualities of soma resemble those of cannabis. Another theory suggests that soma is actual brew from multiple plants, just as ayahuasca brew is made. The preparation of soma as described in the scriptures is a similar process to that of brewing ayahuasca. Whether soma existed, was a mushroom, plant, or combination of all, the

Ancient Indian practices that speak of this mixture is still mystifying to this day and is what intrigues many individuals to visit the area and learn more.

Ololiuqui and the Ancient Aztecs

The rivea corymbosa plant has many traditional uses in Aztec culture and can still be found in use much in the same way among the natives in Mexico and South America. The rivea corymbosa plant is a flowering plant, or twinning herb, that has a slender green stem and blossom of white, blue, or purple. The seeds of this plant are round and either brown or black in color, and it is the seeds that often get much attention for their unique properties, though the whole plant would be used to make different ointments and serum for spiritual and psychic potential. Many of the tribes that use this plant for its powerful effect settled in the mountain regions where it was remote and isolated and would not be scrutinized by Christian views.

During spiritual ceremonies, the priest of the tribes or the area would consume the ololiuqui mixture. They would then enter into a state of what appeared to be delirium. It was in this state they supposed were able to receive messages from divine beings or from those who have crossed over. The priest would talk of the vision he was seeing and the hallucination he saw which would often be terrifying and chaotic.

When spoken about in the many texts written in the tribes at the time, ololiuqui is said to be not only highly regarded in spiritual terms but also in medicinal use as well. Many tribes used it to help alleviate pain, stomach issues, and healing wounds. The healing powers of this plant were said to be of divine influence; this divinity is what these tribes believed made the plant effective at curing many ailments.

The Aztec Sacred Mushroom

There is mention of Teonancatl, translated to mean 'sacred mushroom' in ancient Aztec scriptures and throughout their history. Not much is known about the mushroom though it can probably be assumed that it possesses similar properties to many of the other psychedelic mushrooms found all over the world. While many texts and documents mention the mushroom in the Aztec culture, little attention was ever given to it. It wasn't until Gordon Wasson took part in one of these religious ceremonies that more attention was brought to the use and effects of the mushroom.

Ceremonies and rituals involving these mushrooms can be dated before Christ by almost 1000 years. The mushroom would typically be consumed during feasts or religious ceremonies. Tribe members would be overcome with visual sensations, act intoxicated, and feel energized. While the mushroom was primarily used for religious purposes it was also administered by doctors of the tribe. It was suggested that these mushrooms could supply tribe members with psychic abilities in which they would not only be able to better identify what was causing their ailment but also how to treat and cure what was causing them distress.

The use of these drugs in other cultures often points to religious purposes. Since the effects of these substances had such an impact on those who used them, many cultures believe these effects could have only have been inflicted by a godly power. In a sense, the use of these substances for many spiritual and religious ceremonies was to bring one closer to God, and for many, this is exactly the effect they had.

The Government's Views on Psychedelic Use

When psychedelic drugs first made their way to research labs and therapist offices they were viewed as a breakthrough in the medical field. Patients were seeing immediate relief of depression, anxiety, and PTSD symptoms. Clients were opening up and talking through their traumas with great easy and honesty to truly heal from the inside out. But, just as quickly as they came about they were pushed away. A short time after psychedelic drugs were providing benefits to patients who suffered from psychological disorders, they also became a mainstream recreation drug among the younger generation. Soon, this beacon of light around psychedelic drugs was turned off and psychedelic use was looked at as a rebellious and dangerous activity.

Shortly after LSD made its public appearance, government officials created a classification system that categorized drugs based on their effects and dangers. Psychedelic drugs were quickly added to the Schedule 1 category, clearly indicating that these drugs had no medical value, and were simply highly dangerous. Yet, other drugs which were far more dangerous like morphine and cocaine were categorized as Schedule II drugs. Congress has full control of the classification system under the Controlled Substances Act.

Once the United States began to classify their drugs, other countries did the same which resulted in the UN Drug Control Conventions also creating a classification system for drugs, and they also placed psychedelics in the most dangerous category. Stricter drug policies were adopted by many more countries, including Iran and China.

How do Government Agencies Regard Them Today?

Today, many governments are beginning to change their opinions on psychedelic drugs. In 2001, Portugal became the first country to abolish the penalties in place which criminalized drug possession (Reynolds, ND. Why Were Psychedelics).

In the United States, psychedelic drugs have an extremely negative reputation. They are considered highly dangerous substances and are banned or illegal in most of the country.

Chapter 5:

Different Types of
Organic Psychedelics

Organic psychedelics are some of the most well-known psychedelics. They can often be found all over the world in different climates and are used for a variety of reasons. Even though they are organic, these psychedelics are strictly regulated despite their benefits.

Psilocybin Mushrooms

Psilocybin, known as magic mushrooms, is an organic psychedelic which consists of over 180 different mushroom types. These mushrooms often have a long thin stem with a cone cap and can resemble a number of poisonous mushrooms. This can make consuming them dangerous as it is difficult to be certain if you are consuming the psychedelic version or not. Currently, they are included as a Schedule I substance and therefore illegal in the United States.

While these mushrooms are deeply rooted in Mesoamerica cultures dating well beyond the 15th and 16th centuries, it wasn't until 1955 that magic mushrooms made their way to the young generation of America. Although Albert Hofmann was isolating the psilocybin compound to use in his LSD compound, it was Gordon Wasson who publicly told of his experience with magic mushrooms. Wasson published articles of his psychedelic experience, which caught the attention of Timothy Leary and Richard Alpert.

By 1971, however, psilocybin was placed in the Schedule I controlled substance category and was made illegal in the United States. It is also illegal to grow or possess in most other countries as well.

The effects of magic mushrooms can range from person to person and are often less intense if used repeatedly in a short time frame. This psychedelic tends to be a milder psychedelic with a significantly lower potency rate than LSD. The effects tend to last for about 6 hours depending on the dose.

Psilocin affects the serotonin receptors and sensory receptors which is why they are commonly known for their synthesis effect on individuals, where colors can be felt and music vibrations are seen. Many will go through a trance-state where the user knows they are awake but feels as though they are dreaming. Most of the intense effects of magic mushrooms will occur between one to two hours after consumption. During this time, the user may go through a stage of intense emotions that can feel overwhelming or out of their control, which is what can cause slight panic or paranoia. When one begins to resist these emotions, they can experience a bad trip but if one just lets these emotions flow and run their course, the experience can be quite beneficial. During this process, though it can be frightening for some, the user will begin to simply accept what is occurring and enter into a more relaxed state of mind.

Once in this relaxed state of mind, the individual will often see the world from a different perspective. Many individuals can easily confront difficult feelings or thoughts they tend to avoid, and clarity is then brought to them. Individuals will often feel more at peace and connected to those around them.

Psilocybin mushrooms can be ingested a number of ways, either eaten raw, cooked, or brewed to create a tea. Though the taste may be unfavorable to many they can easily be consumed with other food items to mask the taste. Once ingested, the user will often experience:

- An increase in emotions

- A trance-like state

- Synesthesia

- Loss of time

- Change in heart rate (increase or decrease)

- Change in blood pressure (increase or decrease)

- Tremors

- Restlessness

Most individuals who consume psilocybin mushrooms tend to experience positive changes both during and after their experience. Individuals who have had experiences with psilocybin report having gained a more positive outlook on life and have more ease forming a more meaningful connection with others.

Dangers and Warnings

When taking mushrooms there is a risk of experiencing a bad trip. These trips can result in the user feeling extreme paranoia or engaging in non-typical reckless behavior. The most commonly reported negative effects of consuming magic mushrooms were dilated pupils and nausea.

Aside from these effects, which in almost every occurrence will go away and the person will return to their normal state of being, there is no other documented research that claims that consuming psilocybin mushrooms will or do cause any serious effects on one's health or mental wellbeing.

Peyote

Peyote is a common cactus primarily found in the desert in the Southern United States and Northern Mexico areas. It is an organic psychedelic that has been a part of many Native American traditions and rituals for centuries. As a Schedule I controlled substance it is illegal to grow, sell, or possess the plant, though some exceptions are made when the plant is used in religious ceremonies among Native American tribes.

The mescaline compound in Peyote is what gives it its psychedelic effects. The small buttons pulled from the top of the cactus are typically chewed either raw or dried. They can also be ground and smoked with tobacco or filled into a capsule to be swallowed as a pill. The buttons can also be brewed into a liquid for consumption. Peyote is described as having a bitter taste.

Hallucinations are caused by the substance mescaline found in the cactus which affects the serotonin receptors of the brain. The senses are elevated and often visuals are highly distorted and vibrant. The intensity of the effects will range greatly depending on the dose as well as the user's own desired expectation from consumption. The effects will also be more intense if taking peyote while consuming alcohol or some form of stimulant.

Effects of peyote can last for many hours. Usually during the first one to two hours the individual may experience slight discomforts such as chills, body sweat, and nausea. The peak of the effects tends to occur around four hours after consumption and will then begin to fade. The whole experience can last up to 12 hours or more. The most common effects of Peyote include:

- Euphoria

- Hallucinations

- Loss of time

- Increased awareness

- Relaxation

- Weakness

- Sweating

- Loss of appetite

- Dry mouth

Dangers and Warnings

Some of the most common negative effects that can occur while taking peyote include:

- Increased heart rate

- Increased blood pressure

- Numbness

- Severe nausea

- Vomiting

- Anxiety

- Panic

- Paranoia

While there is not much research involving peyote, some long-term effects that can occur include:

Persistent Psychosis: The user may feel extended periods of paranoia, mood disturbances, inability to think clearly, and continual visual disturbances. These effects will continue even when not on peyote.

Flashbacks: Some users report having flashbacks of their experience while on peyote, these are more likely to occur for up to a week after a peyote experience but can also occur for up to a year after.

HPPD: Hallucinogen Persisting Perception Disorder is a rare occurrence that can cause flashbacks, hallucinations, and visual disturbances well after an experience with peyote and can negatively affect your normal life (Buddy, 2019).

Continuous long-term use can lead to a tolerance of the drug, resulting in the users to require more and more each time they experience it. Long-term use can cause individuals to experience psychological withdrawal symptoms that include depression and dysphoria.

Pregnant women should avoid taking psychedelics in general but especially peyote since it can have negative effects on the fetus.

Ibogaine

Ibogaine is an organic psychedelic that has been a focus for addiction treatment around the world. Ibogaine is extracted from the Iboga plant and other Apocynaceae plant species; the highest concentration is found in the root bark. As mentioned earlier, this plant, native to most West African Nations, has a long history in the babongo tribe. The people first noticed the effect of the plant's roots when the animals that had recently consumed the roots would begin to act in a wild and strange manner.

While it is a Schedule I controlled substance in the United States, some European countries, Canada, and Mexico use it regularly as an opioid addiction treatment. Most uses of these psychedelic drugs tend to be non-recreational (The Essential Guide to Ibogaine, ND).

In small doses, one may feel restless or feel like they don't need sleep. The substance affects various neurotransmitters in the brain and helps increase serotonin levels. Some of the first side effects one experiences after taking ibogaine includes the inability to control muscle movement. For this reason, ibogaine is best taken where you can lay down or remain immobile during the experience, which can last for at least 24 hours up to as long as 72 hours.

The first four to eight hours of the experience will be the most intense. Individuals can expect to be flooded with past memories that they view from a panoramic perspective in a dream-like trance. Hallucinations can occur but more often individuals will pass through space visually as opposed to experiencing the typical visual or noise hallucinations.

After the first eight hours, one tends to experience what is referred to as an "evaluation phase" where one will still be presented with an array of memories but instead of floating through them they observe and reflect on them. During this time, many wish to experience this in silence or at least with a little noise or interference. This process can last up to 24 hours after first consuming ibogaine.

During the last phase of the ibogaine experience, which can last for up to 72 hours, is where the individual begins to become aware again of their immediate surroundings. They begin to regain control over their movement and may even feel more energized.

Many individuals state that for weeks they have a deeper sense of awareness of themselves after the experience. They tend to face their daily lives with a new perspective and are more in tune with their emotions and how they react in situations. While the experience is often life-changing, many who have gone through it agree it isn't the most pleasant experience they have ever had.

Dangers and Warnings:

Studies have shown ibogaine can have negative effects on the heart, causing rhythm problems. Ibogaine contains a complex enzyme that is similar to various chemicals in the body, which is what can cause negative reactions when taking it. Those with heart conditions or complications should refrain from taking ibogaine. Additional negative effects from this psychedelic include:

- Decrease in blood pressure

- Slower heart rate

- Paralysis

- Seizures

- Anxiety

- Trouble breathing

- Vomiting

There have been reports of death from using ibogaine, though these have been looked at as being caused from pre-existing heart conditions or because of interactions with other medications the individual was taking or on at the time of ingesting the ibogaine. Taking ibogaine itself is not reported to cause death.

Ayahuasca

Ayahuasca is an organic psychedelic obtained from the Banisteriopsis caapi vine located in the Amazon, Ayahuasca is well-known among the South American tribes and Indigenous people of the Amazon for its healing benefits. It is often brewed and infused with additional Amazonian plants and used for a number of spiritual ceremonies and rituals. Banisteriopsis caapi vines contain MAOI inhibitors.

Ayahuasca is created when the B. caapi leaves are brewed along with Psychotria Viridis plant leaves. The brew contains the MAOI inhibitors THH, harmaline and harmine, which increase levels of serotonin. When combined with the effect of DMT, one experiences a prolonged period of intense hallucinations. The brew affects serotonin activity in the emotion and introspection areas of the brain.

Most individuals will fast for at least 12 hours prior to taking ayahuasca to avoid negative side effects that can be caused by common foods. The effects of ayahuasca can be felt within the first 30 minutes after taking it which often consists of unpleasant stomach aches, sweating, and nausea. The hallucinations that occur often come about rapidly which results in individuals feeling a brief moment of intense fear or anxiety. After the first intense wave of hallucination, they taper off and come and go through the remainder of the experience. Visual disturbances are common for individuals to experience where objects will appear to move faster, patterns change, and there would be an increase in brightness of lights. These disturbances occur whether the eyes remain open or closed. Noise perception is also altered, making many sounds and noises more noticeable and clear.

The thought process of someone on ayahuasca becomes more specifically focused and give the user more clarity on the subject matter they are thinking of. Many individuals will experience intense emotion throughout the experience, often resulting in a dream-like state.

Those who take higher doses of the psychedelic can expect to feel as though they are traveling through time, have out of body experiences, and experience euphoria. The whole experience tends to last four to six hours but for many, this shorter experience brings about a heightened awareness and personal growth.

Dangers and Warnings

Individuals should avoid eating dairy and consuming alcoholic beverages and chocolates when taking ayahuasca as they can cause negative side effects such as diarrhea and nausea.

Negative side effects that can occur while on ayahuasca include:

- Elevated levels of diastolic blood pressure

- Increase heart rate

- Vomiting

- Anxiety

This psychedelic experience can bring about intense emotional feelings of despair and helplessness. Those who already have a mental health disorder should use precautions when taking ayahuasca in larger doses.

N-Dimethyltryptamine (DMT)

N, N-Dimethyltryptamine, or DMT, is an organic psychedelic drug. The compound is common in a variety of plants and animals but is more often extracted from the leaves of the Psychotria Viridis plant, which are native to Central and South America. It is classified as a Schedule I substance, making it completely illegal in the United States.

The white powder can be inhaled as a vapor or smoked, it is often combined in a brew to create ayahuasca, and it can slowly be injected or snorted. This psychedelic does not tend to affect a specific group of receptors in the brain but often affects many or most at the same time.

One notices the effects of DMT almost instantly - effects occur within just a few minutes and peak very quickly, then they fade away over the next 45 minutes. The whole experience tends to only last for about an hour. The experience may be brief but can be significantly more intense than those you would experience on other types of psychedelics.

An individual will often experience intense visual or auditory hallucinations resulting in a loss of time and space. The intense effects are said to take users to different worlds or periods of time. One of the most notable effects of consuming DMT is the spiritual effects in can bring on.

If consumed as a brew to make ayahuasca, the experience will last much longer, typically about four to six hours.

Dangers and Warnings

While DMT is considered to have the least number of side effects compared to other psychedelics some of the negative effects can be uncomfortable including:

- Change in heart rate

- Change in blood pressure

- Chest pains

- Increased irritability

- Pupil dilation

- Rapid eye movement

- Nausea

- Diarrhea

- Vomiting

Serotonin syndrome can also be a common negative side effect of taking DMT. This can bring on additional side effects such as:

- Confusion

- Lack of muscle coordination

- Headache

When DMT is taken at a high dose, individuals are a greater risk of suffering from more serious side effects such as:

- Seizures

- Coma

- Respiratory arrest

Unlike many other psychedelics, DMT tends not to have a tolerance concern even though it can be easily abused due to the intensity and psychological impact the hallucination can cause.

Salvia divinorum, Salvia

Salvia is an organic psychedelic that comes from the Labiatae plant that grows in Central and South America, and can also be found in southern parts of Mexico. This plant is closely related to the mint family. The leaves of this plant are chewed or the juice from the leaves are extracted to create a drink. Dried Salvia is smoked or inhaled. The common street names for this psychedelic drug are Magic Mint and Sally-D.

It is not classified under any of the schedule control substance categories in the United States, so many states are free to regulate on their own terms. Albert and Anita Hofmann along with R. Gordon Wasson are believed to be the first to document their experience with Salvia.

The leaves of the plant are typically dried and smoked or the salvinorin A compound is directly extracted from the leaves. It can also be chewed or consumed as a tincture. Unlike most of the other psychedelics listed, salvia does not affect the serotonin receptors. Instead, it bonds with kappa-opioid receptors which cause sensory disruption and hallucination.

When smoked or inhaled, the effects of salvia can come on rapidly, usually within seconds and then decline over the next 30 minutes. If chewed, the effect may not occur until up to 20 minutes and the experience can last for about an hour. Many of those undergoing a salvia experience will often begin to notice a tingling sensation and become more aware of their body. Typically, one will experience a clearer train of thought, but when higher doses are consumed, one may instead experience a lack of awareness. Additional effects one can expect from a salvia experience include:

- Increase in visual perception

- Merging with objects

- Hallucinations

- Uncontrollable laughter

- Disconnect with reality

The most notable effect salvia has on individuals is its significant alteration of visual perception. Most people are attracted to this psychedelic because of the effects it can have on the individual psychologically. Salvia also causes individuals to experience a loss of ego where they can explore the inner depths of their consciousness unregulated.

It is advised that one take salvia with a person they can trust who will remain sober through the process. Individuals using salvia are recommended to remain lying down as due to the loss of control of body movement individuals can accidentally harm themselves.

The salvinorin A compound of saliva reduces the release of dopamine while on it and therefore it is unlikely that addiction is possible. Salvia also tends not to have a tolerance build up among users.

Dangers and Warnings

The most common negative effects of salvia include dizziness, chest discomfort, and uncontrollable movements. Because of its psychological effects, individuals can experience a traumatic trip when taking salvia.

Cannabis, Marijuana

There is much debate on whether cannabis or marijuana falls into the psychedelic drug category or not. Cannabis is more so considered a depressant and a stimulant but does not clearly fit into any one type of drug category. It does possess some psychedelic qualities as it can cause hallucination, tranquility of the mind, and has the ability to enhance mood, though it primarily affects signals between the body and the brain.

The hemp or cannabis sativa plant is where Marijuana is produced from; this refers to the dried seeds, leaves, and stems of the plant.

This psychedelic, unlike some of the others, tends to affect much more than just the brain. While mood is often altered, many of the organs in the body are also affected by the chemical compounds in cannabis. This drug is most commonly smoked but can also be inhaled as a vapor, found in a capsule, brewed, or used in baked goods such as brownies.

While cannabis was placed as a Schedule I controlled substance, medical marijuana is not required to be regulated by the government. Medical marijuana can refer to either the whole marijuana bud itself or the components that make up marijuana such as THC or CBD. There are nearly 120 different substances that can be found in marijuana.

THC is what gives marijuana its psychedelic properties. This substance can have an effect on one's mood, brain receptors, appetite, and senses. When this drug is smoked, the THC enters the bloodstream quickly and therefore can affect the brain immediately.

When consumed, it takes longer for the THC to be absorbed by the body and therefore the effects may not be noticed for an hour or two after consumption. THC has similar qualities to the cannabinoids naturally produced in the body which are responsible for sending out signals to the nervous system and are responsible for the functioning of memory, concentration, coordination, perception, thinking, and movement. When THC enters the body, the natural cannabinoids become disrupted.

Some of the effects one may notice after smoking or ingesting cannabis include:

- Relaxation

- Slight hallucinations

- Happiness or euphoria

- Increased energy

Dangers and Warnings

The stimulant properties of cannabis can cause negative effects on an individual psychologically. Those who use cannabis regularly put themselves at a greater risk of anxiety, depression, and experiencing schizophrenia. Those who use cannabis for a long period of time may develop brain function issues as well.

Additional negative effects of cannabis use include:

- Dizziness

- Relaxation

- Tiredness

- Loss of short term memory

- Poor motor skills

- Dry mouth

- Nausea

- Paranoia

- Hallucinations

- Rapid heartbeat

Because of marijuana's ability to delay response to outside stimulants or situations one should not drive after smoking or consuming marijuana.

Frequent cannabis use can lead to addiction or dependency. Those who tend to use marijuana regularly may experience withdrawal symptoms if they suddenly quit using it. Symptoms of withdrawal will begin the second of not using marijuana and can include:

- Increase in irritability

- Stomach aches

- Loss of appetite

- Insomnia

- Anxiety

These symptoms can last for a few weeks and individuals may have difficulty sleeping for longer than a few weeks.

Ololiuqui

Ololiuqui is a plant native to Mexico. The flowers of an ololiuqui plant range from white to blue or purple, but it is not the flowers that give this plant its psychedelic properties. The seed of an ololiuqui plant contains a substance closely related to that found in LSD. D-lysergic acid amide (Ergine) is an organic psychedelic substance that was also discovered by Albert Hofmann, who synthesized LSD. It is listed as a Schedule III controlled substance and is fairly easy to come across.

Ololiuqui has long roots in South American culture. Documents and texts have uncovered a number of stories that describes people's experiences while taking ololiuqui. Most of the stories describe intense hallucinations that are often terrifying and disturbing. Transitions of these tribes suggest that when serum was created from the plant the individual would obtain psychic abilities.

Tribes would traditionally use ololiuqui as a diuretic to cleanse the body and it was also thought to have healing powers when used on wounds and bruises. The Ancient Aztecs would create a potion in order to create an ointment using all parts of the plant. The roots, stem, and leaves also contain psychoactive properties though at a much lower potency.

When used traditionally, fifteen seeds are ground and brewed in liquid for a few hours and then consumed, one can also chew the raw seeds. To bring on a hypnotic state, the seeds were traditionally mixed with mescal or aguardiente. In western culture, it is more likely that one will use up to one hundred seeds to experience its full effects. One can expect a fairly low to moderate experience on ololiuqui seeds. The user will enter a dream-like state with vivid visuals.

For the first four hours, one can expect to experience increased feelings of apathy. This disconnection from one's feelings is accompanied by intense visuals. Light appears brighter, colors are more vivid, and things look more exciting yet peaceful. After this visual stage, the individual will begin to settle into a more relaxed state. Many describe this as being sedated or hypnotized, where they are aware of their surroundings yet lost in some other train of thought.

Dangers and Warnings

The negative side of chewing on the seeds of this plant is that it always comes at a cost of great discomfort. Those who have tried ololiuqui seeds all report feeling intense nausea, stomach pains, and vomiting. These negative side effects usually increase and intensify when more of the seeds are chewed or consumed.

There have also been a number of reports where individuals have ended up in the hospital after consuming ololiuqui seeds.

Individuals should use caution with the type of seed they take. While these seeds are fairly easy to find in many local and chain stores they are not all the same. Keep in mind that many seeds can be treated with certain chemicals which can be poisonous when humans consume them.

Chapter 6:

Different Types of Synthetic Psychedelics

There are a number of both synthetic and organic psychedelics that have been studied or have intrigued researchers and non-researchers alike. Each psychedelic is unique in its own way, providing individuals with varying levels of experiences and side effects. Synthetic psychedelics mimic the effects that most organic psychedelics exhibit but to varying degrees. While the most well-known synthetic psychedelic is LSD, a number of others have been created in the hopes of one day utilizing them for the treatment of various health conditions.

LSD

Lysergic acid, or LSD, is one of the most well-known of synthetic psychedelic drugs. It is a synthetic psychedelic that was grown from ergot, a type of mold found on rye bread. It is considered a controlled substance but is illegal in the United States, though many people take it recreationally and socially.

Users will often experience visual or sensory disruptions, a change in thought patterns, heightened emotions, and often a new awareness or perspective on specific things during an acid trip. Many feel a deeper connection to themselves, nature, the universe, and feel spiritual during and after an acid experience. Those who embrace unpredictability, explorations, and excitement will find taking acid an enjoyable and rewarding experience. Those who on the other hand who have a hard time with the unexpected will often have an unpleasant experience.

LSD can make one extremely emotional which can often be overwhelming and uncontrollable, though this is all dependent on the mood and the environment in which the individual takes the acid. The most common effect of LSD is visual distortions. Many users see swirling patterns, overlays or geometric outlines, sizes of objects are magnified, and other objects tend to take on a life of their own by moving or "breathing". There is often an increase of synesthesia, where sensory perception gets tangled which makes the viewer believe they can see sounds, hear colors, and feel smells.

Auditory, tactile, olfactory, and gustatory hallucinations can also occur. With these different types of hallucinations, one can hear, see, feel, smell, or taste things which are not actually there and these hallucinations can come and go throughout the trip. While a number of distortions, hallucinations, and sensory perceptions can all occur at the same time, which would otherwise cause individuals to panic, many LSD users have the understanding that these are all the effects of the drug.

LSD often has the ability to change one's outlook on themselves, the world, and a number of other areas in one's life. Many users admit that they have experienced a change in their previous beliefs about themselves, what matters to them, and who they are. These changes can be both positive or negative. Many notice they gain a deeper understanding of others as well. They feel more enlightened or spiritual, but they can also feel like life has less meaning, obtain a negative outlook on people, and can begin to alienate themselves more from the world around them.

One does not begin to notice the effects of LSD until almost an hour after taking the drug and this effect can last for up to 12 hours after taking it. Because of the effects one has while taking acid, this length of time can feel even lengthier. The effects of LSD seem to be more intense within the first few hours but the hallucinations and distortion begin to gradually wear off.

Dangers and Warnings

Aside from experiencing a bad trip on LSD, there are other serious concerns that one should be aware of before taking LSD. Other side effects of LSD can include:

- Rapid heart rate

- Increased blood pressure

- Sweating

- Hyperthermia, where the body temperature rises to an alarming rate which can cause kidney and muscle damage

- Dehydration

- Personal safety concerns

It is important to never wander by yourself when you are taking LSD, especially if you are having a difficult time handling the intense emotional or sensory effects. You should always be present with at least one person not taking a psychedelic that you can trust and feel comfortable with. They will be able to remind you that you are safe and that it is just the effects of the drugs in case you do have a bad trip.

It is also important to stay hydrated during your trip, but don't drink excessively. Acid trips can cause one to sweat excessively which can increase thirst. This thirst can be so intense that it can be difficult to quench; this can result in water intoxication, where too many electrolytes are pushed through the body, resulting in the brain being unable to function properly because of excessive water consumption. Those taking acid should avoid consuming caffeine, alcohol, or other substances that can further alter or impair their mental state or mood. Taking LSD can be a tiring experience and many who take it find it difficult to sleep or eat during the final hours of the trip and even afterward.

Risk of addiction is low when taking LSD, though the user can develop a tolerance to LSD when taking it constantly for days at a time. It is often the hallucinations that people become more addicted to as opposed to the overall feeling when taking the drug.

MDMA, Ecstasy, Molly

3,4-Methylenedioxymethamphetamine, or MDMA, is a synthetic psychedelic and is simply the name given to its chemical compound. It was first created in 1914 and was supposed to be used as an appetite suppressant, but by 1980 it was a common and favored drug among festival goers and within club life. MDMA goes by a number of names, including E (Ecstasy) and Molly. Molly refers to the powder form of the drug whereas Ecstasy refers to the pill version; the street versions of the compound often contains less MDMA or none at all. While still considered a hallucinogenic, most experiences do not result in hallucinations or anything nearly as intense as those experienced on other psychedelic drugs. This drug tends to increase alertness and is often more of a stimulant rather than a hallucinogen.

MDMA is commonly taken as a pill or snorted. Effects of the drug are often felt within an hour of ingesting it and the whole experience can last for about six hours. MDMA affects serotonin, dopamine, and norepinephrine levels, which are responsible for regulating mood, appetite, and sleep.

One can expect to be more affectionate while on MDMA because of the increase in serotonin levels.

One may experience a range of psychological effects such as:

- Euphoria

- Extreme contentment

- Increased empathy

- Self-confidence or ability to be oneself

One can expect to experience a loss of time while on MDMA, heightened moments of sensitivity, especially to touch, and an increase in energy levels.

Those who have MDMA experiences report having deeper relationships with others.

Dangers and Warnings

Ecstasy and Molly are often viewed as dangerous club drugs with a number of reports of users ending up in emergency rooms. This is often more likely due to the impure amount of MDMA found in these drugs and other substances that are often mixed with them to create the street drugs.

Other negative side effects that can occur when taking pure MDMA include:

- Inability to concentrate

- Anxiety

- Chills

- Dry mouth

- Imbalance

- Difficulty with leg movement

- Tightening of the jaw

- Decrease in appetite

- Increase thirst

- Restless legs

- Inability of the hypothalamus to regulate body temperature as well

- Hyponatremia (drinking too much water)

MDMA impairs the body's ability to regulate its body temperature which is where most of the serious risk derives from. When taking MDMA in a crowded, overheated club the risk increases significantly as increased energy levels and movement from dancing will further increase body temperature to dangerous levels.

Some negative side effects may also occur for up to seven days after an MDMA experience which primarily can affect your mood, causing some symptoms of depression. These effects are often due to taking an impure dose of MDMA.

MDMA can also become an addictive drug and therefore many users will experience mild to severe withdrawal symptoms that can last for up to a week after use. These symptoms can include:

- Inability to sleep

- Increased irritability

- Anxiety

- Depression

- Inability to concentrate or focus

- Impulsivity

When taken in high doses, MDMA has been shown to cause nerve damage to brain cells. MDMA can also cause an individual to perform abnormal behaviors that can result in more dangerous choices.

Phencyclidine, PCP

PCP was briefly tested in the 1950s as an anesthetic. It had an effect on the brain receptors as well as the glutamate neurotransmitters. It quickly became a recreational drug in the 1960s but had serious side effects on users. PCP comes in a variety of forms including tablets, capsules, and liquids or crystal powder. Angel Dust is the common street name for this powder but may also be referred to as Love Boat or Peace Pill.

It is considered a dissociative psychedelic.

Those who take PCP can expect to have hallucinations, but they vary greatly from those experiences with many of the other psychedelic drugs mentioned. These hallucinations can cause schizophrenic episodes that give users an invisibility complex. This often results in them thinking and behaving in a manner that is not and should not really be acted on, such as jumping from buildings or off bridges or trying to outrun trains. Many users also experience having convulsions after taking too much PCP.

Dangers and Warnings

Severe hallucinations are common when taking PCP. These hallucinations will often cause users to act out of character and exhibit destructive and severely dangerous behaviors. Many individuals who take PCP report to self-mutilate while on the drug. This is one of the rare psychedelics that can be addictive and can cause symptoms of withdrawal.

When taking high doses of PCP, individuals run the risk of:

- Seizure

- Coma

- Death

If you decided to take PCP you need to be sure to avoid taking it while also consuming other mind-altering substances such as alcohol or benzodiazepines as this can further increase the risk of coma.

Ketamine

Ketamine is a legal drug most often used as an anesthetic, but can also cause hallucinations and other side effects commonly associated with psychedelic drugs. It is a dissociative synthetic drug which was first used in the 1960s. Ketamine was the result of trying to create a safer alternative anesthetic to PCP. It is often found as a powder or in capsule form. Liquid Ketamine can also be obtained and injected or cooked to create a powder that is then snorted. The most common street name for this psychedelic is Special K.

Ketamine, unlike the other psychedelics on this list, is classified as a schedule III controlled substance, meaning it is legal to administer and receive the drug in medical settings.

Ketamine experiences are often less intense and last for shorter periods of time, although the effects are quite similar to PCP. Many have an enjoyable experience on Ketamine and often have an out of body experience with feelings of floating or gliding through time and space. One can experience hallucinations though they tend to only last briefly, or experience a total detachment from the sense and gain enlightenment in deeper areas of their own mind. One will often feel a sense of euphoria as well as experience an increase in happiness and feelings of total relaxation.

Dangers and Warnings

When taking significantly high doses of Ketamine one can experience what is called a "K-Hole" (Hartney, 2019. K Hole). This occurs when the user is unable to move their own body or even interact with people around them. The user becomes completely immobile and is often unable to speak. A K-Hole experience can be compared to a coma state where hallucinations take over reality, leaving the individual to feel completely powerless and fearful. This experience can be difficult to emerge from and feelings of disconnect can last for prolonged periods of time.

Some experiences of a K-Hole can result in long-term psychosis. Additional serious side effect of ketamine can include:

- Seizure

- Heart failure

- Brain damage

Ketamine can be tasteless and is regularly used as a date rape drug.

Dextromethorphan, DMX

This synthetic psychedelic is a common ingredient in a number of cough syrups and cold medicines. The most common street name for this drug is Robo. In small doses, there are no serious effects of DMX but when consumed in higher quantities there can be a range of side effects.

Considered a dissociative psychedelic, DMX can have similar effects as Ketamine. When higher quantities are consumed, one can experience hallucination, enter a trance-like state, or enter into a euphoric state. A typical DMX experience can last for up to eight hours.

DMX is typically consumed in liquid or gel capsule form, as it is often consumed by drinking or taking over-the-counter cough medicines. Pure forms of DMX can be obtained which come in a powder or liquid form where it will need to be snorted or injected.

The most common side effects of DMX include:

- Increase in auditory perception

- Increases in visual perception

- Hallucinations

- Increase in excitement

Dangers and Warnings

The most common negative side effects of DMX include:

- Nausea

- Vomiting

- Constipation

- Fatigue

- Anxiety

- Dizziness

- Confusion

- Irritability

- Chills

- Increased heart rate

- Stomach aches

- Paranoia

- Difficulty speaking

- Seizures

Death has also been reporting when taking DMX, and consuming alcohol with DMX significantly increases this risk. Additionally, those who regularly ingest DMX in high doses can suffer from long-term psychosis.

2C-1, Smiles

2C-1 is a synthetic psychedelic drug that is a combination of stimulants, hallucinogens, and amphetamines, and it is often referred to as Smiles or bath salts. It is a fairly new synthetic drug which was created by Alexander Shulgin in 2000. For close to a decade, little was heard of this new drug Smiles, which was a popular street drug that was being secretly passed around to teenagers and young adults. Until it made headlines in 2011 when two teenagers apparently died after taking Smiles, not much attention was ever given to the drug. Smiles is a Schedule I controlled substance according to the United States category system.

Smiles is often obtained as a white powder or pill and it can either be snorted or mixed with foods for consumption. As a hallucinogen and stimulant, one will experience the effects of both these components. The effects can be similar to experiences with LSD and ecstasy.

The most common effects one can expect to experience while on Smiles include:

- Visual hallucination

- Audio hallucinations

- Relaxation

- Euphoria

- Increase in empathy

Dangers and Warnings

The most common negative effects one can expect to experience while on Smiles include:

- Anxiety

- Panic

- Fear

- Increase in blood pressure

- Inability to concentrate

- Memory impairment

- Nausea

- Vomiting

- Seizures

While there is little scientific research on 2C-1, one can assume that many of the negative long-term effects would be similar to those of both stimulants and hallucinogens, which can include:

- Depression

- Heart problems

- Kidney damage

- Psychosis

- Dependency

- Addiction

- Death

Because there is so much uncertainty around the negative effects of this drug, and because it is often bought illegally on the streets, one needs to use extreme caution with this drug. It can be incredibly easy for this drug to be mixed with a number of other harmful substances to increase its street value. Since it has intense hallucinogenic effects, many individuals believe that it is not likely that they will overdose on this drug. Because of its stimulant component, it is highly likely that overdose can occur. Blood pressure can also be significantly increased to the point where they reach a deadly level.

Chapter 7:

Common Household Items You Didn't Know Were Actually Psychedelics

Surprisingly, you may have consumed a psychedelic already and never even realized that you did; there a number of psychedelic items you might find in your own kitchen. While these items have the potential to give you the same effects as the previously mentioned psychedelics, it is not advised that you actually try to consume them to have a psychedelic experience. In order to feel the effects of the following psychedelics, you will most likely have to consume a large quantity, which not only is unsafe but can cause unwanted sickness.

Nutmeg

Nutmeg is a common spice used in many baked goods and can easily be found in most home spice racks. Nutmeg contains myristicin with is a compound that will give similar effects that you would experience while on LSD (Georg, 2019). Myristicin is also the compound that MDMA was supposedly structured after. If you could take a high enough dose to bring about an experience you could expect it to last two or three days and filled with hallucinations. Negative side effects that you could potentially experience include:

- Diarrhea

- Nausea

- Vomiting

Additionally, consuming high amounts of nutmeg can lead to heart or nerve problems.

Morning Glory

Morning glory flowers can be found on many front porches or backyards and these flowering plants fall into the same family as ololiuqui. Morning Glory may also be called Heavenly Blue or Pearly Gates. They contain LSA, which is what gives them the potential to provide you with a psychedelic experience. The seeds, which can be easily found in many nurseries and stores, are often chewed, though it would take up to at least 100 seeds to be able to feel the effects. Often times, more is needed.

Individuals should use caution with the types of seeds they use. While morning glory seeds are fairly easy to find in many local and chain stores they are not all the same. Keep in mind that many seeds can be treated with certain chemicals which can be poisonous when humans consume them.

Sage

Sage, or more specifically Sage of the Diviners or See's Sage, is a plant that is typically grown in the forests in Mexico. This plant has been used for years as a part of spiritual ceremonies. The leaves of the plant contain a high concentration of salvinorin, which is where the psychedelic effects come from. The leaves are often dried and smoked or brewed into a tea. The plant is illegal in the United States and it is not likely that you have this type of sage in your pantry.

Hawaiian Baby Woodrose

Hawaiian Baby Woodrose, also known as the elephant creeper, is a vine that produces large flowers and is common in India and also grows in Hawaii, the Caribbean, and Africa. Like the Morning Glory, this plant also contains LSA. One can expect to have less intense experience with Hawaiian Baby Woodrose but can obtain more mental clarity and focus.

Cough Medicine

Most over the counter cough syrups contain DMX. If you consume enough of the cough medicine you could experience hallucinations and a euphoric state that can last up to six hours. However, consuming the wrong dose of cough medicine can be fatal because of the additional ingredients in the medicine. Despite the risk, and often terrible taste, cough medicine is often the most misused item in households across the United States. It is highly recommended that you do not drink cough medicine unless needed to treat a cough or cold.

Chapter 8:

The Effects of Psychedelics

Psychedelics will affect individuals in varying ways, this is often called a "trip" or "experience". It is because of these experiences or trips that psychedelics have such an appeal. They can be viewed as an escape from the world, a pathway to understanding, or simply a way to have a good time. While the youth of the 1960s are viewed as using these drugs as a way to simply have a good time, they actually had a greater understanding of their effects, one of which those who had not had the pleasure of experience are unable to grasp.

Those who have used psychedelic drugs notice the effects tend to influence three main components:

Sensory - Users tend to feel a heightened awareness of their senses. Individuals will often see more vivid colors, richer textures, and sound is resonated more deeply. There are also instances where one can become more aware of their own body and limbs. It is not uncommon for shapes and objects to appear distorted or that one may be able to feel sound and hear colors. This effect on sensory input results in one feeling as though time has slowed down or stopped.

Emotional - The emotional effects of psychedelics cause the person to feel extreme joy, anger, love, terror, and any other emotion one may feel. These extreme emotions are linked directly to the mood of the user at the time of taking the psychedelic. Users can often feel more than one of these emotions at the same time. When taking a psychedelic, the user can also be more aware of other people's expressions, gestures, and behavior and this often magnifies them, which often results in these extreme emotional experiences.

Environmental - The overall mindset and environment the person is in when they take the psychedelic will also have an effect on their experience. If the person is anxious, paranoid, or even depressed when taking a psychedelic this will often result in an unpleasant experience for the user. If the individual is open-minded and believes that the experience will be enjoyable, the experience often becomes an enjoyable one. Along with state of mind, if the environment is too noisy, busy, or unsupportive, which also clashes with the state of mind the person has, this can also result in a negative experience. Again, if they are in a fun, relaxing setting then this will often result in a more pleasant experience.

Good Trip. Bad Trip

When taking psychedelics, one can often have a good experience or trip, or an unpleasant, terrifying experience or bad trip. Each drug will offer users varying experiences. The dose also has an impact on what type of experience or trip you will have. Often times these are not the only factors that will determine what type of experience you will have. Who you are with, your own expectations, and your environment has a direct impact on the type of experience you will have.

The comparison of a "good" trip versus and "bad" trip is often made as a good dream or a bad dream. Since the effects of many psychedelic drugs can make the user feel like they are dreaming or in a trance, this seems to be an accurate way of identifying what a good or bad experience is. When one experiences a good trip they often feel pleasant, the world looks more beautiful, life is more wonderful, being around other people is more meaningful, and deeper connections are made. Understand that one can have a terrifying experience at first because of the intensity of heightened senses and hallucinations. However, this will often subside once one remembers that what they are experiencing is because of the drug and accepts that these terrifying visuals will often transform into more pleasant and enjoyable ones. Just because you may have to confront unpleasant feelings or visuals does not necessarily equate to your experience being bad. Many factors can come into play that will result in a bad trip.

On the other hand, a bad trip can result in feeling overwhelmed, intense fear, the world being viewed as harsh, cruel and ugly, life seeming painful and sometimes meaningless. Other people can often be viewed as superficial and unbearable. These kinds of bad trips can bring on extreme negative thoughts such as suicidal thoughts. When one experiences a bad trip they are more at risk of having an accident while on the psychedelic drug. This is due to the lack of understanding they have of their experience. What they are experiencing is so intense that they are doing everything they can to escape from it, which is not possible until the effects of the drug wear off. Another negative experience is when the individual obtains superhuman beliefs while on a psychedelic. This can often result in the person believing they are able to do things that would otherwise be impossible, such as flying or running faster than a speeding train. This can result in horrific and serious injury.

Psychedelics can give individuals the sense that time is standing still. While having a good trip this is a welcomed feeling, but when having a bad trip this can only intensify the negative feelings. Many individuals think the horrific experience will go on forever and will never stop. Having this type of experience can cause the person to feel deep despair. Additionally, a bad trip can occur when the person suddenly has opposite views of people or situations. They may look at the people around them as close friends that they can trust and then suddenly while on the psychedelic they may become fearful and untrusting of the same people around them. This can put the person in a dangerous position as they will often want to try to get away from the people they are with, and it is never wise to let someone on a psychedelic go off by themselves.

A bad trip can often result in extreme panic, out of control behaviors, and even violent acts. This is often the portal psychedelic drugs present and is often the reason why so many have a negative opinion on psychedelic drugs. While you cannot one hundred percent prevent or even stop a bad trip from occurring, if it does, there are ways you can make a bad trip less intense.

- It is best to lay down if you are having a bad trip. Sitting or standing can often cause hallucination to be more intense and cause more visual disturbances. Laying down puts you in a more relaxed position which can help alleviate negative feelings and visuals.

- Playing calming music throughout the experience can help keep the environment calm.

- Have a trusted friend stay with you through the experience. They can help reassure you during the negative experience that it won't last forever and that you are safe.

Often times it is easy to avoid having a bad trip if you properly prepare for the experience. You will learn about this in the 6 S' of the Psychedelic Experience section in this chapter. What also must be noted is that there are varying levels that one can experience when taking a psychedelic drug. The higher the level the more risk there is to have a bad experience, but it is also at the higher levels that many experience the most profound breakthroughs and feelings of enlightenment. Additionally, one must keep in mind that each psychedelic drug will present its own set of stages or phase you will go through. Often times the most intense hallucinations and visuals will occur near the beginning of the experience then will subside and one often enters a state of bliss. There will still be visual disturbances but they are counteracted with a new sense of enjoyment or peace.

The Levels of Psychedelic Experience

What constitutes the level of intensity when it comes to having a good trip or a bad trip? Though it is difficult to thoroughly explain just what one experiences while on psychedelics or the true quality of the experience, Timothy Leary did an adequate job outlining the levels one may go through when taking psychedelics.

Level one:

This level is experienced when taking very mild psychedelics such as cannabis. One will experience a change in mood, subtle changes in sensory perception, typically with sound. Mild psychedelics at this level will often show a change in communication between the left and right side of the brain, this is usually an increase in communication between these two areas.

Level two:

This level is experienced when high levels of a mild psychedelic like cannabis is used or a very low dose of a moderate psychedelic like psilocybin mushrooms or peyote. At this level, the users will begin to see more vivid colors and distorted visuals even when the eyes are closed. The thought process and emotions begin to see an effect where creativity is increased and emotions begin to change; usually emotions become more intense, whether it is joy or sadness, and a new perspective is being gained on the outer and inner world.

Level three:

This level is experienced when taking a normal dose of a mild psychedelic like psilocybin or LSD. At this level, the psychedelic experience often involves distorted patterns, figures, and images; this is experienced whether the eyes are closed or open. One will often feel a change in their energy levels and may begin to gain a new perspective on life. A trance-like state is possible and out of body experiences can occur.

Level four:

This level is experienced when a higher dose of mild psychedelics and stronger psychedelics are taken. At this level, the user begins to experience intense changes in sensory perception as well as a disconnect with time. The user will often see objects begin to move, hallucinations begin to manifest, out of body experiences being regular occurrences, and achieving deeper spiritual enlightenment. Most users who experience this level of the psychedelic experience have admitted to gaining a clear perception or a greater sense of knowledge. Level four is where many can begin to have transformative experiences.

Level five:

This level is achieved when high doses of psychedelics are taken or DMT is consumed. The quality of this state varies greatly compared to the other levels. The user becomes consumed by the visuals they experience. As the highest level of the psychedelic experience, one can feel completely transformed or cleansed. One is often plunged into a void-like space where they view the world through new, yet dysfunctional glasses, and they run through the cosmos having an out of this world experience. They report to having incredible speed in which they can take on the shape of other objects and will encounter mythical creatures.

Level five is the most extreme experience that one may encounter while on psychedelics, and while it does sound tempting to encounter each of these levels, what is experienced individually can be the opposite of each description.

The 6 S' of the Psychedelic Experience

Set, setting, substance, sitter, session, and situation all impact the type of experience you will have when taking a psychedelic. If you take time to properly consider these 6 factors you can better increase the chance of having an enjoyable and beneficial experience. According to The Third

Wave article that outlines the 6 S' for a good psychedelic experience, they can be approached as follows:

Set

Set refers to your mindset. When you take the time to understand what your expectations and desires are through the psychedelic experience you are more likely to have that type of experience. The user should take the time to properly prepare their mind for the experience by understanding what they truly think about psychedelic experiences, what goals they attend to achieve, and what things they want to learn, resolve, or understand more. Being able to clearly answer these questions in regard to your own expectations of your psychedelic experience will help you have a more open and relaxed mind.

Setting

The setting in which you will have the psychedelic experience is a vital component to having an enjoyable psychedelic experience. The best option for the setting of your psychedelic experience should be either an uncluttered room that allows you to remain comfortable and relaxed or a familiar setting that is set in nature. If choosing an indoor setting keep sharp objects out of sight and fill the space with pillows and blankets. If choosing an outdoor setting bring pillows and blankets along with you so you can lay down comfortably. You can also choose a location that provides the option of both indoor and outdoor spaces.

Other things to take into consideration with settings is incorporating music; music which can help enhance the experience and promote an atmosphere that is enlightening. Classical music, chants, instrumental piano songs, or drum focused songs are ideal. It is best to avoid music that has words, which can become a distraction.

Substance

Substance involves knowing how much of the psychedelic you need to take to reach the level of experience you are expecting. Every psychedelic is different and the amount you will need to take varies; the experience you wish to have will also have an impact on how much you take. For those wishing to simply improve their productivity and trigger creativity than a microdose is strongly suggested. For those wishing to have a more enhanced experience that includes slight alteration to sensory receptors and an increase in hallucination, a more moderate dose may be required. Those wishing to have a full-blown psychedelic experience may consider taking a larger dose but do so with caution.

Sitter

The sitter refers to the person who will act as a guide for the psychedelic experience. If possible, you will want to share your expectations with this sitter prior to the experience to understand how to better achieve what you desire. The sitter will remain sober for the experience and is there as a support person. While not always necessary it is highly recommended to choose a sitter who has experience with psychedelics and can therefore assist you better if your experience does not go so well. You can also ask a close friend who you fully trust to serve as a sitter but be sure to make them aware of what things to be concerned about and how to properly handle the situation for the full duration of the experience.

Session

A session refers to how long do you want the experience to last. When considering the session, you need to consider the various phases each psychedelic experience will also present. There are typically six stages or phases you will go through in one session; the length of each stage varies depending on the type of psychedelic.

Situation

The situation refers to what occurs after the psychedelic experience which can often be weeks or months that follow the experience. During this time period, it is wise to sit and consider what you actually learned through your experience. Often these will be things that you will have a new perspective on or better clarity over. In the weeks that follow a psychedelic experience, many individuals take into account what really matters in their lives and where they want or need to make changes.

How Do Psychedelics Affect the Brain?

The main reasons why psychedelics interest so many in the healthcare industry from psychologist to researcher, is because of the way they directly affect the brain. While many drugs and treatments aim to do the same, psychedelics can have a longer lasting impact than what is seen or felt instantly.

While psychedelics clearly have an effect on perception and the senses, this is due to the effect it has on multiple areas of the brain, like with neurotransmitters and neuronal structures. When these neuronal structures are affected, this results in a change in a person's thought patterns, behavior, and feelings.

The brain is composed of dendrites which grow dendritic spines, and through the spines, signals are received, processed, and sent out. Neurons are composed of these dendrites and spines as well as synapses. When a brain is not functioning properly, often caused by a mental disorder or illness, these dendrites stop growing or simply shrivel up. This is a common effect in those with depression, post-traumatic stress disorder (PTSD), anxiety, and other psychological disorders. When someone takes a psychedelic drug, there is an immediate reaction that triggers the growth of these dendrites and spines (Olsen, 2018). This immediate growth of the neurons is believed to be the result of a psychedelic compound's effect on a protein called mTOR used in cell growth.

The binding abilities of many psychedelic drugs can also have long-term positive impacts on personality traits. Individuals who have taken psychedelic drugs tend to score higher in areas of openness, or their ability to show more gratitude and enjoyment from new experiences. Even individuals who only took psychedelic drugs once in their lifetime have either stated that the experience was the most life-changing aspect of their lives and that the long-term personality changes greatly improved their quality of life (Specktor, 2014).

Public Opinion on Psychedelics Being Used as New Medical Treatment

With increasing concern of the opioid epidemic occurring in the United States as well as many other countries around the world struggling with their own form of addictions among their population, effective treatment is a top priority. This significant increase in addiction and overdose reports leave the general public desperate for a truly effective way to eliminate the crisis.

As new understanding and reports are being made public and shared there seems to be a shift in the public view on psychedelic drugs. They are beginning to be viewed as an effective way to not only help treat addiction but a number of other health conditions. The once negative reputation they gained in the early 70s shifted towards a reputation that could ultimately improve quality of life for many.

The picture previously painted during the Nixon campaign portraying drugs as dangerous and a serious public concern for safety is shifting to one that sees the flaws and deception in the picture painted. While these psychedelic drugs can be used recreationally there is little risk of them ever becoming a concern for addiction. When practiced in a safe and responsible way the drugs have a positive impact on those who choose to undergo a psychedelic experience.

Over the past few years, more studies are being conducted and the public is becoming more educated on the effects of psychedelic drugs. There seems to be a strong urge for lawmakers to make changes to the current drug policies to allow these drugs to be used for medical purposes and treatments. The 'War on Drugs' is no longer a concern, as many of the psychedelic drugs classified as Schedule I substances have more restriction on use than many opioids, which are listed as Schedule II or III substances, even though opioids are known to have addictive qualities and negative effects on users.

A more concerning factor for the public is that many addiction treatments, mental health treatments, and long-term medical care management is not only costly but ineffective and can take years to see progress with. Psychedelic drugs are being viewed as a more effective and immediate solution to managing a number of disorders that are often left untreated.

Many countries, aside from the United States, have already begun to take advantage of the beneficial use of psychedelic drug use for treatments. Some countries have even completely decriminalized drugs and have seen significant drops in overdose and mental health reports. More countries are allowing for in-depth research and studies to be done to demonstrate the effects of psychedelic drug use and treatment. The United States is falling behind in many of these areas as they have yet to make changes to the declassification process or allow for such testing to be conducted without researchers going to rigorous steps to gain approval.

Chapter 9:

Scientific Testing

From the 1950s to the 1970s, hundreds of tests and trials were conducted on the effects of psychedelic drugs to treat depression and addiction. While a majority of the tests had displayed exciting results, a ban was placed on psychedelic drugs and abruptly stopped what could have been a major turning point in medical history. Research and findings that involved psychedelic drugs had to be done secretively or in hidden areas of the world.

MAPS

Funding for medical research around psychedelics was halted when the Controlled Substance Act was put into effect in 1970 (Reynolds, 2018). Being guaranteed permission to even possess a small number of psychedelic drugs for continued research and testing was made nearly impossible then. This left many medical professionals at a loss as to how to continue the promising research they had spent a decade conducting.

In 1986, the Multidisciplinary Association for Psychedelic Studies, MAPS, was created to find a way to help fund research and spread information around psychedelic drugs. The organization is a non-profit which relies on memberships to help educate the general public and encourage a new understanding of the health benefits of psychedelic drugs.

Since it was first founded, the organization has assisted scientists in funding and gaining approval for research and studies to be conducted on the safety of psychedelic drugs and other controlled substances. The members work closely with government agencies such as the FDA and EMA to set up protocols and guidelines required to move forward with the studies. They can be credited with helping with a number of studies done on MDMA, LSD, and psilocybin and the benefits they provide for individuals who suffer from PTSD, anxiety, depression, cluster headaches, and addiction.

The organization also sponsors a number of medical education ceremonies, lectures, publications, and more to keep the general public aware of the progress and results from testing and studies conducted. This organization has become a vital component to the continual research that takes place involving psychedelic drugs and their benefits.

The Beckley Foundation

The Beckley Foundation was formed in 1998 by Amanda Feilding. The organization, which originated in the UK, focuses on drug policy reform as well as continued research on psychedelic drugs. The foundation works with their Scientific Programme and in collaboration with leading scientists and experts to gain a better understanding of the effects that psychedelic drugs have on the human body. This is done through clinical trials and projects and has played a vital role in understanding more about the toxicity, chemical compounds, and specific reactions that psychedelic drugs have on the brain.

Medical Testing and Findings

Previous papers and documents are being reviewed once again to see where modern scientists can pick up where the scientists of the 60s and 70s left off or were forced to stop. With improvements and major advancements in technology, scientists are able to better understand just how psychedelic drugs impact the brain and act as an effective treatment for many disorders. Brain scans are able to highlight exactly which areas of the brain are affected by psychedelics and scientists are able to make hypotheses as to what compounds or chemicals in psychedelics are activating or affecting those areas of the brain. These new advancements can open doors for scientists to better engineer synthetic drugs that can be just as effective as organic psychedelics but without the unwanted side effects or intense experiences.

When studies were first being conducted there was still a number of things that scientists need to understand about psychedelics. To begin, many of the initial trials administered higher doses of these drugs, which would result in intense experiences for participants. Not much was done to study the full effects and benefits of what smaller doses of these drugs could provide for patients before the ban was set on all psychedelic testing.

With the assistance of MAPS, psychedelic testing was still taking place, though it was often done with a much slower and drawn out process. In the early 2000s, new generation scientists began to look into the findings of these earlier tests and trials that involved psychedelics. More and more people began to see just what potential these drugs possessed and began conducting trials and tests of their own. Many of these tests and trials were random, scientists would often have to travel to different countries to record scientific evidence that psychedelic drugs should be looked at as a serious alternative that can effectively treat various disorders. As the years pass, more research is being done, more scientists are pushing for Congress to reconsider the classification levels of some psychedelic drugs, and in many other locations around the world that is what is beginning to occur.

Studies and Trials on LSD

Early findings

LSD was first tested to see how effective it would be to help reduce the risk of hemorrhaging during childbirth. Albert Hofmann was attempting to create a drug that would control blood flow from lysergic acid. He modified the lysergic acid compound 25 times until he finally set the project aside as all the versions were not as effective as he intended them to be. LSD-25, as he called it, sat on the shelf of the laboratory for nearly five years before Hofmann would revisit the sample. After accidentally absorbing one of the LSD compounds into his skin, Hofmann began testing on himself to understand the full effects of what he had created. During his first experience, he unknowingly administered himself a large dose and experienced the psychedelic properties. Hofmann found himself feeling refreshed and energized after the first test was completed and other researchers in the same lab began to test the effects of LSD-25 on animals.

Aside from Hofmann, Werner Stoll was one of the first individuals to be administered a low dose of LSD in a psychiatric setting. What was discovered was that LSD was able to help aid the young man to confront repressed memories in a more relaxed and controlled manner. After this initial trial, LSD was given the name Delysid and marketed as a way for psychiatrists to help patients uncover repressed emotions and feelings.

LSD encouraged scientists to rethink what the underlying cause for certain disorders, like schizophrenia was. When LSD was being looked at as a psychiatric tool, researchers revisited the idea of trying to understand what the biochemical origins were that could cause schizophrenia. Experiments first done on LSD were believed the drug was able to put users into a state of psychosis, as users exhibited visual distortions and obsolete views of reality when on the drug.

In 1953, LSD was first used in psycholytic therapy for therapeutic purposes in England. Observation of patients who underwent this type of therapy showed they were more open and comfortable about talking about repressed thoughts or memories. Unlike other treatments methods, LSD allowed patients to communicate logically through the session as opposed to in a state of delirium. When LSD was administered in a low dose, therapists could guide patients to dive deeper into understanding and in turn work through the attachment they had with the negative feelings, thoughts, or events that troubled them.

In 1954, psychedelic therapy was first used in Canada to help alcoholics become sober. Unlike in England where LSD was being used for the therapeutic benefits, in Canada, therapists believed if they could cause alcoholics to have such a negative experience they would be too fearful to drink again. Patients were given high doses of LSD but instead of having the horrific experience therapists hoped and tried to create, patients instead had pleasant and enjoyable ones (Williams, 1999). Researchers changed their approach and began to guide patients through the LSD experience and point out to them how it related to their drinking. From these trials, LSD was no longer looked at inducing a psychotic state, and research began to take a new path. When word got around about psychedelic therapy, other countries began to implement the practice as well. Prague, for instance, began to use this form of treatment for heroin addicts with great success.

In 1960, LSD was known as a popular recreational drug, but research showed some of the negative effects that could be caused if LSD was not used properly. Studies were published trying to give LSD a negative image to help reduce the recreational use of the drug, and in 1962, regulations were beginning to be put in place that would require approval for additional drug testing to be conducted. LSD was no longer being supplied to therapists to use in sessions and a year later, much of the research that was being done on the drug had been stopped (Williams, 1999). Though LSD showed great promise and benefits in therapy sessions, no further studies could be done once the classification schedules were formed in 1970.

For the next ten to twenty years, there were apparently no human studies conducted involving LSD, but many animal studies were. Though the use of LSD is no longer legal in the United States, or many countries around the world, a few countries in Europe still used psychedelics in therapy sessions.

Microdosing

LSD is one of the most favorable drugs to use in microdosing - a process where individuals take a significantly lower dose of a drug over a short period of time. Because LSD has shown capabilities of improving mood, reducing depression symptoms, encourage creativity, and stimulate cognition. Studies that focus on how LSD, through microdosing, can affect one's mental health and brain activity are currently being conducted.

What can LSD possibly treat?

The studies conducted on LSD have shown great promise that LSD can be an alternative and effective form of treatment for those suffering from:

- PTSD

- Depression

- Anxiety

- Drug addiction

- Alcohol addiction

Trials conducted in London in 2016 reported that LSD could potentially change the thought patterns of participants. Participants of the study had no history of mental illness. Each person was given a low dose of LSD and participants reported feeling more open, optimistic, and happier. These effects tended to last for at least two weeks. This study indicates that LSD can be ideal for treating depression (LSD as a, 2018).

Studies and Trials on MDMA

Early Findings

When MDMA was first being used among psychiatrists there was little to no testing on the effectiveness of the drug. While it showed the benefits of aiding psychiatrists in getting patients to open up more easily it was a much more popular drug used for recreational purposes. It was banned for a while in 1985 but in the early 90s was approved for a human trial to determine its effectiveness on reducing severe pain in patients as well as its effectiveness in psychotherapy sessions (MDMA, ecstasy abuse, 2017).

MDMA was one of the psychedelic drugs used in the CIA project MKUltra. During the 1950s, the CIA was looking into the effectiveness of psychedelic drugs being used as a form of weapon and mind control. It is reported that only non-human subjects were used to test MDMA which gave researchers the first glimpse of MDMA toxicology studies.

In the late 1980s the MAPS organization was conducting further toxicity and human safety studies regarding MDMA. In the 1990s the FDA approved for a study to be conducted using a double-blind placebo to show if MDMA could be of value in the medical field. In 2004, another study was approved to research the effectiveness of MDMA to treat PTSD. The results of this study showed that MDMA could be used to help eliminate PTSD symptoms and that the results were long-lasting. Additional trials also showed the effectiveness of MDMA along with assisted psychotherapy which showed just as exciting positive feedback.

In 2016, new studies began to expand on MDMA benefits in additional therapy sessions. MDMA-assisted Cognitive Behavioral Conjoint Therapy is also being studied, but no publications of the results have been made public yet. Through this study, it might be shown that this type of therapy will help couples communicate more openly in therapy, especially when one of them suffers from PTSD.

In 2014, MAPS obtained approval to further MDMA and its effectiveness to help treat anxiety, specifically social anxiety present in adults on the autism spectrum. Additional clinical trials and studies are also being conducted to further understand the effects MDMA has on the brain and there is much hope that the result will open up new doors to future research and eventual implementation of MDMA to treat a wide range of disorders.

Reports showing an increase in empathy and a reduction of fear from individuals who took MDMA encourage researchers to look more into how MDMA can be used by psychologists to allow patients to open up more comfortably during the therapy session. This is being specifically researched when it comes to PTSD treatments.

MDMA increases a lot of activity in the brain. It not only increases the chemical levels of serotonin, dopamine, and norepinephrine which results in more activity between the neurons in the brain, it also triggers the release of corticosteroid and oxytocin. The increase in these stress hormones and bonding agents is the unique effect that MDMA provides and where many antidepressants fall short.

What can MDMA possibly treat?

The studies conducted on MDMA have shown great promise that MDMA can be an alternative and one of the most effective forms of treatment for those suffering from:

- PTSD

- Social anxiety in autistic adults

Many clinical trials and studies are being conducted to see what other conditions MDMA can help treat, but for the past 20 years, PTSD and anxiety have been the main focus of studies that have been approved.

Studies and Trials on Psilocybin

Early Findings

While LSD was being focused on for psychological effectiveness, psilocin and psilocybin were newly discovered psychedelic substances. They were isolated by Hofmann, were tested and shown to have similar side effects as LSD, and then integrated into therapy treatments.

In 2000, efforts were made to reintroduce psilocybin research. The process for gaining approval can take years of effort, and in 2016, the Beckley/Imperial Research program was able to make the data gained from a recent study regarding psilocybin public. The study was conducted to show the effectiveness of psilocybin to reduce depression symptoms among individuals who have resistance to other forms of treatment. More than half of the participants showed no signs of depression in a one-week follow-up. Three months after the initial treatment, which included psilocybin, over 40% of individuals still showed no signs of depression (Psilocybin, Our research with, ND).

In 2016, a studied that involved cancer patients who were suffering from anxiety and depression were given a single dose of psilocybin or niacin along with psychotherapy. There was an immediate and noticeable reduction in anxiety and depression symptoms among the group who received the low dose of the psychedelic. At the follow-up assessment almost 7 months after the initial dose, more than half of the participants still showed a significant reduction in depression and anxiety symptoms. They also had a more positive outlook on life, an increase in spirituality, as well as were more accepting of death.

Additional studies are being conducted to show the effectiveness of psilocybin-assisted psychotherapy to help treat smoking addiction and other addictions.

What can Psilocybin possibly treat?

The studies conducted on Psilocybin have shown great promise that psilocybin can be an alternative and one of the most effective forms of treatment for:

- Those suffering from OCD

- Anxiety in cancer patients

- Those suffering from Depression

- Those who have a smoking addiction

Studies and Trials on Ayahuasca/DMT

Ayahuasca brew combines the components of two plants, which is why it is such a powerful psychedelic. Ayahuasca on its own without the boosting power of DMT can cause individuals to have intense experience just the same, but for a much shorter time period. Many tribes around the world use ayahuasca in order to have enlightening and spiritual experiences.

Technology has granted researchers a better understanding of just how ayahuasca affects the brain through brain scans. These scans revealed the ability of ayahuasca to regrow neurons in the brain, which leads many researchers to believe that this psychedelic can help aid in repairing cells that are damaged in the brain.

Studies have shown the effectiveness of ayahuasca psychotherapy on those who suffer from various types of substance abuse due to psychedelic therapeutic components.

Ayahuasca typically brings one to a level where they are able to observe thoughts and feelings without passing judgment on themselves. Those who suffer from depression, PTSD, or anxiety may benefit from having this type of experience. More studies are being conducted to show just how this type of mindfulness brought on from ayahuasca use can be an effective way to reduce symptoms of depression, anxiety, and PTSD.

More research still needs to be done to fully understand the effects ayahuasca can have on an individual and the risks must be weighed against any of the possible positive findings. While it has shown promise to help individuals in a therapeutic setting, there is just not enough data to understand just how beneficial this psychedelic can be. Additionally, the brewing of ayahuasca is a very intricate process that takes much time and focus to do. While studies show valuable information in regard to how it can stimulate cell growth, there may be other psychedelics researchers should focus more of their attention on.

What can ayahuasca possibly treat?

The studies and research conducted on ayahuasca have shown great promise that ayahuasca can be an alternative and one of the most effective forms of treatment for those suffering from:

- PTSD

- Anxiety

- Depression

- Alzheimer's disease

- Dementia

- Substance abuse

This psychedelic still has years of testing and research to go through before there is any chance of it being used as a viable alternative to already existing treatments.

Studies and Trials on Mescaline/Peyote

Much of the research and testing of peyote and its compound mescaline are done with the assistance of Native American tribes, which was hard to gain their trust as most tribes did not like the idea of scientists disrupting their daily life. These tribes are the exception to the illegal use of peyote as they use it for spiritual and religious rituals. One study involving 200 participants, aimed to show how effective peyote could be for treating alcoholism. The results of this study showed that peyote could help individuals resist the urge to drink for up to six months.

Brain scans show that serotonin receptors are activated when taking peyote and will often activate other areas of the brain as well. Studies report that those who have taken peyote will often see an improvement in the ability to solve problems and retain information.

What can mescaline/peyote possibly treat?

The studies conducted on mescaline/peyote have shown great promise that mescaline/peyote can be an alternative and one of the most effective forms of treatment for those suffering from:

- Mild forms of mental health disorders

- Depression

Studies and Trials on Ketamine

Ketamine was already used as an anesthetic when psychedelic drugs had begun to be researched on. Many research and studies have been conducted to prove the effectiveness of ketamine to help treat depression.

Ketamine was looked at for its ability to produce fast-acting antidepressant symptoms to patients who had found other treatments and drugs ineffective. In 2019, a nasal spray was approved by the FDA to help treat individuals who had treatment-resistant depression. This nasal spray contains esketamine, which is a compound derived from ketamine. Studies done prior to approval showed that participants who suffered from depression typically saw immediate improvements either the same day or the next day in their depression symptoms. These effects seemed to last about two weeks.

Unlike many other antidepressants which have to be present in your system to have an effect, the nasal spray doesn't need the esketamine to stay in your system. Since it triggers activity in the brain, once it's done, it doesn't have to remain in your system.

Studies of this new antidepressant are still new and data collected only goes back for about a year, so there is still plenty to learn about its effects. However, data has shed new light on the psychedelic health benefits.

What can ketamine possibly treat?

The studies conducted on ketamine have shown great promise that ketamine can be an alternative and one of the most effective forms of treatment for those suffering from:

- Severe depression

- Anxiety

- PTSD

Studies and Trials on Cannabis

Of all the psychedelic drugs, cannabis has probably been the most common and most controversial psychedelic drug. In the United States, many states have set up their own regulation and criminalization method regarding cannabis which could be why there is much controversy around the drug. California was the first state to approve medical marijuana use and later went on to legalize recreational use of marijuana for adults. Though research on cannabinoids in cannabis had already been done well before the 1900s when the Controlled Substance Act was enforced in 1970, cannabis was placed under the schedule I category Cannabis has been used for centuries to help relieve severe pain. Cancer patients had been smoking cannabis and taking Marinol, a drug that contained THC, to help relieve nausea symptoms brought on by chemotherapy treatment.

Cannabis has been a part of history for nearly 5000 years and there is suggested evidence that as early as 400 A.D., cannabis was used for medical purposes. Countries around the world use cannabis for recreational and medicinal purposes, for example, those in Jamaica who have been known to use it to rinse their eyes to help reduce the risk of glaucoma.

Most of the research first gathered on the use of cannabis

was done so by individuals who used it recreationally at first.

Two components of cannabis were of great interest for researchers, THC and CBD. These two components have been researched extensively and scientists have found that THC is the compound that causes psychedelic effects while CBD supplies individuals with pharmacological effects. Research is still being conducted to understand the most effective way to administer this drug to provide patients with the most effective results in the shortest amount of time.

Because CBD does not have psychoactive effects on the user this has been the prime component that has been thoroughly studied.

In 2018, the CBD drug Epidolex was approved to be used to treat rare forms of epilepsy.

Although THC does have psychoactive effects, researchers believe this component can also provide individuals with health benefits. Studies showed that THC can be used to help alleviate vomiting and nausea, especially among chemotherapy patients. Other studies have shown THC to be an effective alternative to help treat chronic headaches.

Research is still being conducted to see how effective cannabis use can be used to help kill off cancer cells. In 2016, there were reports from researchers showing that cannabinoids have the ability to hinder the growth of tumor cells. Because high amounts of cannabinoids can have negative effects on the immune system, this can result in additional cancer cells to grow unnoticed.

What can cannabis possibly treat?

The studies conducted on cannabis have shown great promise that cannabis can be an alternative and one of the most effective forms of treatment for those suffering from:

- Nausea

- Vomiting

- ALS

- Epilepsy

- Chronic pain

- BPS

- Migraines

- Osteoarthritis

- Rheumatoid arthritis

- Fibromyalgia symptoms

- Osteoporosis

- DDD

- Huntington's disease

- Parkinson's disease

- Tourette's syndrome

- Glaucoma

- Hypertension

- Anxiety

- Depression

- Sleep Disorder

- PTSD

- Schizophrenia

- Alzheimer's disease

- IBS

- Cancer prevention and treatments

- OCD

- ADHD

- Chronic Heart failure

- Malaria

While cannabis has shown promise to help treat and alleviate pain symptoms from those suffering from various conditions, there are a number of known long-term side effects that need to be carefully considered. Unlike many other psychedelics, there is a risk of addiction with cannabis.

MKUltra, Government Testing

While scientists were looking at the therapeutic benefits and properties of psychedelic drugs, government agencies were looking at them for the complete opposite reason. In 1953, the CIA began to conduct their own research on the side effects of psychedelic drug use.

This CIA project was titled MKUltra and its sole purpose was to gather information and a better understanding of how psychedelics could be used as a form of mind control. With the country in a constant state of fear of a threat of another war, the CIA was taking drastic measures to prepare if this event should ever occur. There was hope that psychedelic drugs would allow American troops to psychologically torture during interrogations and used them as a form of mind control over enemy soldiers. The experiments conducted through project MKUltra were illegal and used innocent people as test subjects in the

United States and Canada. Extremely high doses of LSD were given out to individuals in hospitals, schools, and prisons, sometimes forcefully and sometimes unknowingly. What the CIA found from these experiments were kept a secret, and most evidence that these experiments ever occurred was burned just before the Watergate Scandal. It wasn't until 1977, however, that project was finally put to a stop.

Additional Research Being Conducted

Research on DOI, 2,5-Dimethoxy-4-iodoamphetamine

DOI is a synthetic psychedelic that was first discussed in 1972. Not much is known about this psychedelic drug, though it has been a highly researched psychedelic. The first reported use was in 1991 by Alexander Shulgin. It is often used to help map out serotonin receptors. DOI presents side effects similar to LSD, though the experience tends to last much longer and can be more stimulating. Research shows that DOIs can promote rapid growth of neuron connectors and can be a promising form of treatment for degenerative diseases such as Alzheimer's disease and rheumatoid arthritis, and other conditions where there is severe tissue damage due to chronic inflammation that could not be reversed.

New Zealand and Mexico are currently the only countries that use Ibogaine as an effective form of treatment for drug addicts. Ibogaine is illegal in most parts of the world including the US and is highly restricted in the UK, forcing many individuals to seek out these treatment resorts as a last effort to kick their habit. The resort can be expensive but is well worth the price. Studies that have been spanned eight years show compelling evidence that with just one dose of Ibogaine, serious addicts can remain sober and avoid withdrawal symptoms which often resulted in their ability to remain sober. The treatment does not come without serious side effects. Nineteen reports of death have been linked to the treatment, but upon further examination, most of these cases had a pre-existing heart condition or liver condition which was more likely the cause.

A study conducted in 2008 might help explain why ibogaine is such an effective form of treatment. In this study, it was reported that the GDNF protein levels in the brain greatly increased when one took ibogaine. This GDNF protein is what helps prevent addiction from developing.

Drug testing is hindered significantly because of the strict ban on psychedelics. While many studies and trial shows promising potential of these drugs it is still unclear if they pose and long-term negative effects. Because psychedelic drugs are so strictly regulated it is nearly impossible to conduct a longer study to understand these effects. What many researchers are trying to accomplish is to engineer drugs that will provide individuals with the same benefits as psychedelics but will be viewed as much safer.

Chapter 10:

What Can Psychedelics Help Treat?

Psychedelics affect the brain in a unique way, which is why researchers are so interested in further studying and understanding these drugs. Because they are able to change the structure of the brain, it makes them a strong candidate as an alternative to treat a number of mental and neurological disorders. Their therapeutic properties can make them highly effective when used with therapy to help treat a number of mood disorders. A great deal of research and clinical trials have already been conducted that show psychedelics can change the way the following disorders, conditions, and diseases are treated.

Depression

Depression is a medical condition where individuals have extreme feelings of loss and suffering. In the past, depression was primarily thought to have been a result of chemical imbalances in the brain, but with advancements in technology and a number of studies, it is now believed that depression is much more than just a level imbalance. Depression doesn't just affect one's mood but can take over one's life by causing the individual to have a loss of interest in activities, socializing, and even living. It affects what you do, how you act, and what you think. Depression can often have serious effects on individuals and their relationships. While there are many treatment options available for depression many can be ineffective or take months or years to see change. Since psychedelic drugs were first synthesized in labs they have been looked at intensively for how they can help treat this disorder.

Psychedelic drugs have been looked at as an effective way to treat depression because they directly affect the ability for neurons in the prefrontal cortex to grow and attach to surrounding neurons. They not only promote the structural growth to the neurons but also function by triggering communication between the new neurons and neurons in other areas of the brain. Ketamine has been one psychedelic that has been shown to provide fast-acting effects on both the structural and functional operations of these neurons. As a result, this has been able to provide those suffering from depression immediate or almost immediate reduction in symptoms.

Using psychedelic drugs like psilocybin allows emotions to come more naturally which then causes those individuals to feel more in control of what they are feeling. They also have a way of reprogramming the brain and can result in those connections that were deeply rooted in depression symptoms to be disconnected, triggering new connections to be made. A number of psychedelic drugs that have been tested show positive results in helping those who suffer from depression, especially those who have depression that has been resistant to other forms of treatment. Ketamine was studied and found to be one of the most effective antidepressant drugs that help trigger an immediate response in the prefrontal cortex. The prefrontal cortex is the area of the brain responsible for emotional control - when someone suffers from depression the neurons become disconnected from the rest of the brain. Ketamine promotes regrowth and new connection to occur between this area of the brain and the disconnected areas.

MDMA, or Ecstasy, has been one psychedelic drug that has shown great potential to treat depression. The drug produces very mild hallucinations and positively affects the enjoyment receptors in the brain. It has also been shown to increase empathy and reduce fear in individuals, which makes them more able to acknowledge what they are feeling and how those feelings are affecting them. Since MDMA is a synthetic drug, it also contains stimulant properties. These properties further trigger the release of serotonin in the brain. Scans have shown that low serotonin levels are a common factor among those who suffer from depression.

Psilocybin has also been researched frequently on its effectiveness in treating depression. This is because psilocybin directly affects the brain's serotonin receptors.

Possible Negative Effects:

The increase in the release of serotonin can cause serotonin deficiency when psychedelic drugs are used in high dosages for long periods of time. These consistently high doses can result in chronic depression.

Mood disorders

Individuals who suffer from mood disorders experience moods that are disconnected from their current circumstances. Mood disorders can range from depression to bipolar disorder and can affect all age groups. Traditional treatment of mood disorders consists of medication, primarily antidepressant and talk therapy. While these treatments can be effective for some individuals who suffer from this condition it can often be a long drawn out process that rarely rids the individuals of the disorder even after long periods of time. For other individuals, these types of treatments are simply ineffective.

It has been shown that the neurites located in the areas of the brain responsible for regulating mood, anxiety, and reward response tend to waste away or die. Communication stops between these areas of the brain, which is what brings on many of the symptoms of mood disorders. Psychedelics have shown the ability to regrow these neurites to restore communication to various parts of the brain.

When psychedelics were first discovered, they were tested and found to be effective as additional treatment for individuals suffering from depression, anxiety, and other mood disorders. While it may still be years away before psychedelics are commonly used in practice, psychedelics have already shown their ability to help those suffering from various mood disorders. Where the issue primarily lies is finding a psychedelic drug that is safe enough for patients to take with them to use in their own home. Researchers are now focusing on engineering drugs that offer the same benefits of psychedelics by triggering the regrowth of neurites, but that do not present other side effects.

PTSD

Post-traumatic stress disorder is a debilitating disorder that can significantly decrease one's quality of life. PTSD is classified as a psychiatric disorder that is often experienced by those who have suffered from traumatic events. Individuals can often relive the traumatic events, unknowingly realizing it is just a memory or past figure they are visualizing in the present moment. Many who suffer from PTSD, especially those who have been in combat, suffer from nightmares, insomnia, uncontrollable mood swings, and erratic behavior. Those who have PTSD are at a greater risk of becoming addicts, having poor relationships, being unable to maintain a job, and depression. Most medication available to treat PTSD is considered highly addictive with prolonged use and often come with a long list of negative side effects.

PTSD is commonly known to affect those who have or are serving in the military. There are nearly 22 reports a day of Veterans committing suicide because of their PTSD (MDMA Therapy Offers Breakthrough. ND). Studies show great promise in the use of MDMA in therapy sessions where patients are able to confront, talk about, trust, and come to peace with the events that caused the PTSD. They also show that patients have breakthrough moments when administered MDMA and show significant progress just after a session or two.

MDMA has shown to have positive effects on those suffering from PTSD. MDMA allows victims to feel more comfortable with confronting the emotions from the trauma they suffered. It gives them a feeling of security and heightened empathy while also decreasing their fear around the events that took place. The calming state of mind one enters while taking MDMA allows PTSD patients to open up about the traumatic events in a way they have been unable and unwilling to do so with alternative therapy and treatment options. Unlike traditional PTSD medication, MDMA has been viewed as a more effective way to get patients to open up and work through the trauma in a much shorter amount of time.

Anxiety

Anxiety is a normal and justifiable reaction to various situations faced throughout the day, certain situations, and is often nothing to feel concerned over. However, for some individuals, anxiety can take over daily life, making even the simplest mundane tasks appear overwhelming and terrifying. Anxiety disorders are a type of mental health disorder where an individual may feel extremely nervous, fearful, or worried without necessarily having a cause. It is an emotion that can become crippling and affect one's life in extreme ways. Like depression, this disorder has been researched to show that the connection in the brain that regulates anxiety is severed or broken. Psychedelic drugs like MDMA, psilocybin, and DMT have shown to help restore and promote growth of new connections.

Additionally, trials are beginning to see how effective psychedelic drugs can be for those who suffer from social anxiety brought on by autism spectrum disorder. Social anxiety is common among adults with autism spectrum disorder and can greatly impair their quality of life. The first trials came back with promising results, showing that psychedelic drugs along with psychotherapy could help reduce social anxiety in these adults as they showed improvement immediately after the first session lasting for up to twelve months following the treatment.

Alcoholism

While many individuals have a few drinks socially or once in a while to unwind, those who suffer from alcoholism or alcohol abuse tend to not know their limits or consistently go past their limits when consuming alcohol. Individuals who suffer from this disorder tend to drink frequently, and often with a disregard for their own safety or well-being. This disorder can end up having negative effects across many areas of an individual's life from their relationships to work or school. The main issue with this disorder is that many who suffer from it are often in denial about the dependency on alcohol or the quantity they actually drink. Alcohol, being an easily accessible substance that can cause individuals to become dangerously intoxicated, can be appealing to individuals because it provides them a legal way to escape from their problems. Many individuals use alcohol as a coping mechanism without even realizing it before irreparable damage is done.

Alcoholism can be a serious condition that is incredibly difficult to overcome. Because alcohol is so easily available, individuals tend to quickly return to drinking despite how many meetings, sessions of therapy, and changes they make. Psychedelic drugs can help individuals cut back and eventually quit drinking altogether. Alcoholics Anonymous founder Bill Wilson was a strong advocate for the psychedelic drug LSD to be used as an effective treatment to help those suffering from alcoholism. Wilson credited his experience with LSD as being what assisted him with overcoming his alcoholism due to its spiritual effects.

Drug Addiction

Drug addiction is an increasing concern that has been affecting thousands of individuals around the world Over 30,000 people lose their battle to drug addiction every year, and that number continues to grow year after year, with little hope of decreasing. In the same way, alcoholism affects the alcoholic, drug addictions severely affect drug addicts. Withdrawals from drug addiction can be incredibly intense, much more so than the often subtler withdrawals of alcohol. Addicts often experience excruciating pain throughout their body, debilitating confusion, and often feel as if they are going out of their mind. For this reason, many addicts try but often fail at staying sober. Similarly to alcoholism, drug addiction is often a go-to escape for many individuals. Recently, the growing number of addicts is due to an addiction to prescribed pain medication that people are no longer prescribed or can afford. This often forces individuals to turn to alternatives such as heroin to relieve pain that is often no longer present but instead is replaced by a need to feel relief.

Ibogaine has been one of the most successful psychedelics to help those battling with severe addiction. Treatment centers around the world that specialize in using ibogaine as a treatment for heroin and opioid addiction as well as amphetamine, alcohol, and cocaine addiction have become more common. Through this treatment, the individual is given a dose of ibogaine, and since the effects of ibogaine can take three days to fully wear off, many individuals never suffer through the intense withdrawal symptoms common in those overcoming addiction.

While ibogaine does not cure individuals of their addition it does make withdrawal symptoms and cravings more manageable. Many individuals who have undergone this type of treatment felt immediate relief from the withdrawal symptoms they were having when they took ibogaine. Many noticed the symptoms and cravings also did not return for a least a week and were noted to be significantly less intense. They often only returned three or more months later when cravings intensified more.

Epilepsy

Epilepsy is a neurological disorder that causes individuals to suffer from sudden convulsions, loss of consciousness, and sensory issues. This disorder is often the result of unusual activity in the brain. In 2018, the first psychedelic drug was approved to treat this disorder. Epidiolex is considered a synthetic psychedelic that contains cannabis compounds and has been approved to be an effective form of treatment for epilepsy. This cannabinoid solution brings relief to those who suffer from rare forms of epilepsy and are resistant to other epilepsy medications.

Neurological disorders

Neurological disorders like Alzheimer's disease, Dementia, Parkinson's disease, Epilepsy and Multiple Sclerosis, to name a few, are all the result of damage to the nervous system. Most of these disorders offer no cure and only treatments and medication can be used to help manage symptoms or slow down the progress of the disorder.

Psychedelic drugs have been proven to have therapeutic effects on individuals and in this sense, can be highly beneficial to those suffering from a neurological disorder. LSD has been tested and reported to leaving individuals feeling more positive about their condition and more accepting of it. This can help these individuals obtain a better quality of life.

OCD

Obsessive-compulsive disorder, OCD, can affect individuals to varying degrees. This condition causes individuals to hyper-focus on unwanted thoughts, feelings, or ideas. This hyper-focus then drives the person to react to these things with repetitive behaviors, actions, or words. OCD is recognized as a type of anxiety disorder which can cause severe manic episodes if the repetitive patterns are interrupted or forced to be avoided. While individuals may acknowledge and agree that the behaviors or thoughts they have are unrealistic or unreasonable they are unable to simply stop them. Treatment for this disorder often revolves around various therapies, the most common being cognitive behavioral therapy. Treatment can often take years to see any progress being made if any at all, and patients often run the risk of suffering from a worse condition brought on by panic and fear.

Individuals who suffer from this disorder often do so secretively. Many of those who suffer from the disorder fear the shame and misunderstanding that is often associated with the disorder. While many television characters portray this disorder a weird and comical trait, the disorder can become highly disruptive in one's life, making it almost impossible to live "normally". Often those who suffer from OCD never try to seek out proper treatment or help.

Psychedelic drugs offer a more effective alternative that can provide the patient with much faster results that last longer. Individuals who suffer from OCD show signs of the 5-HT reuptake inhibitors in the brain being severely affected by the disorder, shown through brain scans. Psychedelic drugs, such as LSD and Psilocybin, affect the 5-HT2A receptors as well as the 5-HT2C receptors which can offer those who suffer from OCD relief or reduction in symptoms.

Quitting Smoking

Though everyone is well aware of the dangers of tobacco use, millions of individuals still smoke. While tobacco use is no longer heavily endorsed and many precautions have been put into place like campaigns designed to reduce the urge for individuals to smoke and regulations being put into place, tobacco use is still the leading cause of individuals being diagnosed with preventable diseases. Smoking is more than just an addiction to the chemicals in the cigarettes, it is also an addiction to the simple act of doing it. One of the main excuses individuals attribute to the cause of them being unable to quit is that they don't know how to replace their smoking habit with something more productive to fill the time they now have. The habit of smoking becomes so ingrained in a person's behavior that breaking the habit is seemingly impossible for many smokers. Add the habit to the unpleasant withdrawal symptoms one has to suffer through that can last for weeks, and it is not surprising why many individuals rarely make it through the first 24 hours before needing a cigarette.

Those who have tried to quit will often exhibit intense mood swings or aggression, nervousness, anxiety, and fatigue. While there are a number of products available to help individuals quit smoking most are ineffective and many smokers return to smoking after just a short amount of time.

Additionally, many of these products have warnings and labels stating the long list of negative side effects, warnings, and concerns. Smoking is a highly dangerous habit that often not only affects the smoker but also those around the smoker.

Psychedelic drugs have shown to be an effective alternative that can help individuals quit smoking. Not only have tests shown psychedelic drugs to be effective but also considerably safer than many products or prescriptions currently available to help individuals quit smoking. Because of psychedelics' ability to bring to light the root of the cause of the addiction they can help individuals truly understand how they have made this habit such a significant part of their life and allows smokers to address the patterns they see in a more open and honest way.

Cancer Treatment

Individuals who have been diagnosed with terminal cancer, or who have cancer in an advanced stage, are often at a greater risk of and do suffer from anxiety and depression. A small study headed by Charles Grob, a psychiatry professor at UCLA, documented the effects of psilocybin on these types of patients. The results showed that the psychedelic allowed patients to better face their fears around death and reduce their anxiety over their diagnosis. This first study was conducted in 2010, then John Hopkins and New York University conducted studies in 2016 that showed the same beneficial results in patients and also showed a decrease in symptoms of depression among terminally ill patients who went through psychedelic therapy. The studies showed an immediate reduction in symptoms of depression and anxiety after the first treatment session which reportedly lasted for up to six months.

The use of psychedelics among patients undergoing cancer treatment doesn't focus on curing cancer or preventing the inevitable, it focuses on assisting those facing the disease to gain a better understanding and acceptance which allows them to continue to live their lives as fully and happily as they can. The trials conducted show that after just one low dose of the psychedelic drug there was a significant improvement in patients and a reduction in symptoms of anxiety and depression.

Chapter 11:

Psychedelic Therapy/Psychotherapy

There are many ways psychedelics can be utilized to help treat patients suffering from many types of disorders. When psychedelics are used alone, individuals can experience significant changes in their symptoms but many patients will still need to consider and require a therapy component that will further allow individuals to fully overcome their conditions and better manage them. Psychedelics can also assist therapy in better treating patients with disorders where they have made little progress with therapy alone.

What is Psychedelic Therapy?

Psychedelic therapy was a widely used form of treatment for many individuals in the 1960s and 1970s before psychedelics were banned and treatment with psychedelics was put to a stop. During this time period, psychedelics held a lot of promise to help treat a number of disorders where other drugs and treatments were ineffective. Now, this approach to treatment is beginning to rise with increasingly greater success rates.

Psychedelic therapy implements the use of low dose psychedelics in a traditional therapeutic setting. This low dose is administered to help patients feel more comfortable with confronting their thoughts, feelings, and past experiences. This method has seen positive impacts on the way therapists have treated individuals who suffer from:

- OCD (obsessive-compulsive disorder)

- Anxiety

- Depression

- PTSD (post-traumatic stress disorder)

- Addiction

- Eating disorders

Through this type of therapy, the psychedelics are utilized as tools and are not considered a cure for the patient's disorder. There are two styles of therapy used when following this approach. Some therapists will administer low doses of a psychedelic during the therapy session. This is done more frequently, usually over a two-week time frame, to allow the therapist to assist the patient as they go through the psychedelic experience. This is referred to as psycholytic therapy and often results in a less overwhelming experience for the patient. In other instances, the therapist will administer a high dose of a psychedelic once or a few times. The psychedelic is taken while the patient stays in a special clinic and is involved in a therapy session before and after the psychedelic experience. The patient is typically advised to take the drug in the evening so the experience runs its course through the night. The staff in the clinic is there as a support team to ensure the patient remains comfortable and calm during their experience. This is considered psychedelic-assisted therapy where the patient goes through a transformative experience while on the psychedelic.

The most common psychedelics used in these therapies include:

- MDMA

- Psilocybin

- Ayahuasca

- LSD

While this type of therapy is not accessible in the United States since the use of psychedelic drugs is illegal, there are many countries that utilize this therapy, such as Mexico, South America, Switzerland, Canada, The Netherlands, and some parts of Europe. There is hope that the United States will make this therapy a viable option over the next few years. Psilocybin and MDMA are the two most used psychedelics for this type of treatment since they are often easier to administer and the effects do not last as long as other psychedelic drugs, making it easier to monitor the patient.

The Benefits of Psychedelic Therapy

Psychedelic therapy has proven to be an effective way to treat difficult disorders. One of the most notable benefits of psychedelic therapy it that just one session can have a major transformation in the lives of the patients. With just a few psychedelic therapy sessions a year, the patient can make a complete transformation in their lives in a way that was never conceivable in the past.

The main reason the therapy can be more effective than many other traditional therapies is that the use of psychedelic drugs gives the patient a new perspective to approach their issues. Patients are able to look at their thoughts and feelings without having any deep connection with them. They are able to finally see them for what they are. They also in a more relaxed state of mind, they are more trusting and more capable of being open to what they are experiencing. This can make talking about the issues they are facing easier for them and give new insight to the therapist. Many mental conditions leave individuals unable to understand their behaviors, thoughts, or feelings, and this makes it even more uncomfortable for them to talk about them or open up about them. Additionally, many of these patients suppress memories or thoughts that need to be addressed in order for them to heal and move forward. Psychedelic drugs open up these doorways in the mind and allow the patient to finally accept what is really going on.

Traditional therapy aims to accomplish the same openness and clear communication in sessions. Often it can take months to have even one small break, and the process can be a long and drawn out ordeal that can actually leave patients feeling as though nothing will ever change. Psychedelic drugs speed up the process of getting to the route of what is really causing the issue so patients can start confronting them and healing from them.

While this treatment is still in the clinical trial period there have been positive results shown in various studies. In one study, 107 patients who suffered from PTSD underwent psychedelic therapy. Nearly 60% of the individuals report to have no symptoms of PTSD just two months are their psychotherapy treatment. MDMA was used in this study and because of the results, the FDA acknowledged MDMA as a possible breakthrough drug to effectively treat PTSD (Bennington-Castro, 2017).

Psychedelic therapy is viewed as a vital tool for those with mental health issues because it allows the patient to explore their own thoughts, emotions, and experiences on a much deeper level. The low dose allows patients to become more relaxed and willing to open up about issues they may have been suppressing for years. Since psychedelics directly affect the biology of the brain's chemistry it is likely that the result will be longer lasting and more beneficial than other forms of treatment that focus solely on emotions.

Doubts Surrounding Psychedelic Therapy

Even though there are promising results from the many clinical trials already conducted, this is not enough to completely sway the doubtful minds of many individuals. Since psychedelics have had a negative reputation in the past and there has been a great misunderstanding to how these drugs affect the brain and individuals in general, there is an increasing concern that the use of psychedelic drugs as a treatment option will only result in a bigger drug epidemic.

There is also concern over the effects these drugs will have on the individual's psyche if they are already suffering from a mental disorder. While the doubts and fears seem justified, the first studies conducted on psychedelics show no signs that these drugs will result in the person forming an addiction. When these drugs were first studied they were studied by administering higher doses. Using lower doses has a milder effect on the individual, and additionally, the setting in which the drugs are administered are highly controlled, which reduces the risk of a negative experience from the patients.

Chapter 12:

Microdosing

Microdosing is not a new practice, as the creator of LSD was known to microdose. Entrepreneurs like Steve Jobs have admitted to microdosing, and even credited his experience to be what led to the simplistic design of Apple products (Lembo, 2019). Many individuals use this practice to help manage depression, anxiety, and other ailments as well as to increase creativity levels and improved productivity. Microdosing simply involves taking a very low dose of a psychedelic multiple times over a short period of time. This allows the user to feel the benefits of the drugs but without the intense side effects when taking a higher dose. Microdosing is also used in the clinical trials of psycholytic therapy, where patients are administered a low dose of a psychedelic drug during therapy sessions.

LSD and psilocybin mushrooms are the psychedelics of choice when microdosing, and individuals tend to stick to a schedule when doing so. It is believed that by taking small doses over a short period of time, individuals will have more mental clarity with heightened awareness. Amanda Feilding, the founder of the Beckley Foundation, has conducted self-reports of the benefits of microdosing and makes it a mission to introduce and teach others about the benefits as well. In the reports, it is suggested that microdosing has a direct impact on one's cognitive and creative abilities (Lembo, 2019).

The goal of microdosing is to alter one's perception, not necessarily to experience hallucinations. The extremely low dose makes this more possible to achieve. In over a week's time, the individual will take a low dose of the psychedelic on the first day, skip two days then take a second dose, skip another two days and then take the final dose on the last day. In order for the process to be effective, one should keep a journal to document and track the experiences, thoughts, and changes they notice day to day.

While there is no specific scientific documentation that showcases the benefits of microdosing, there are many personal stories that have been shared that reveal its benefits. Many of the individuals who practice microdosing report not only being able to alleviate depression and anxiety symptoms but also that they gain a more positive outlook on life and improvement in their mood throughout the experience.

Benefits of Microdosing

Most individuals who admit to microdosing revealed they experienced:

- Improve mood

- Positive outlook on life

- Increase in productivity

- Better focus

- Decrease in depression symptoms

- Regulated mood

Warnings and Precaution to Microdosing

Since there is no scientific research that has been conducted on the benefits of microdosing it is difficult to know if any risks are associated with it. However, from reports that state that regularly using psychedelics in high doses can cause heart damage, it can them be presumed that if one practices microdosing more frequently they could increase their risk of suffering from some form of heart disease. Additionally, figuring out the right dose to take while microdosing may take some trial and error which can result in having a negative experience through this practice. Finally, taking psychedelics too often builds up a tolerance to the effects. This is why microdosing is spread out over a week's time with days in between doses. Building up a tolerance to psychedelics will not necessarily result in addiction but can result in unintentional abuse of the drugs.

Chapter 13:

How Else are Psychedelics Being Used?

While psychedelics are primarily being focused on for being used for medical purposes there are additional ways that one can benefit from psychedelics, even though they may not have a medical condition that requires it. Individuals who are feeling stuck in their life, lack motivation, want to spark creativity, want to feel as though they have a more meaningful purpose, or want to positively impact their quality of life by obtaining a more positive view on the world, can benefit greatly from a psychedelic experience.

In this chapter, you will learn some of the additional ways psychedelic are being used to heal, inspire growth, and bring more compassion and connectivity to the world.

Healing Purposes

There are a number of secretive healing rituals being performed that allows people to benefit from the enlightening effects of psychedelic drugs. These rituals are typically guided by a group leader who encourages individuals to group together in a safe space for the mind-altering journey. Healing rituals and psychedelics are no strangers - for thousands of years, organic psychedelics have been the center of a number of rituals from rites of passage to spiritual and self-discovery ceremonies.

These healing rituals are better known as plant medicine ceremonies, where the facilitator acts a shaman of sorts and ensures the safety and wellbeing of all individuals partaking in the ceremony. Once the full psychedelic experience has come to an end for the participants they gather around to share what they experienced; often times this is through mandala drawings. They also discuss how they can incorporate the lessons they learned and what they experienced into their everyday lives.

While the psychedelic is a main component of these ceremonies this is not done for simple recreational use. In fact, it is often a privilege to be able to take part in one of these underground ceremonies, according to those who have participated. Participants are there willingly because they want to change something in their lives. For many this is being able to control their depression or anxiety, for others, it is to help them overcome a devastating event, and for others, it is to dive deeper within themselves to find a purpose in the life they are living.

But perhaps those that received the greatest benefit out of

these ceremonies are those who struggle with addition. Many individuals seek out these ceremonies a final effort to stay clean and sober. They have often tried every therapy, treatment, or recovery programs available to them but also end up turning back to the substance of choice. After participating in one of these ceremonies many addicts have been able to manage cravings, stay clean, and obtain a new view on life that gives them hope. They often discover through the experience that they no longer have to turn to drugs or alcohol to escape and that they no longer need to run from what drove them to the drugs and alcohol in the first place.

Retreats

The Psychedelic Society was originally founded in San Francisco and has since spread into a global movement with locations around the world. This organization hosts a number of retreats throughout the years in areas where psychedelics are more accepted by society. It provides individuals the opportunity to come together to have a psychedelic experience in a judgment free zone. These retreats are often considered therapeutic and life-changing. Aside from retreats, The Psychedelic Society hosts additional events where individuals can learn about the true scientific benefits of psychedelic drugs. Their mission is to correct and enlighten those who have been misinformed for decades about the use of psychedelic drugs.

Spiritual

Since the first documented uses of organic psychedelics were primarily focused on spiritual or religious ceremonies and rituals, it is no surprise that even today many are using psychedelics for the same reasons. Spirituality is different for everyone and doesn't necessarily refer to organized religion. Many individuals who use psychedelics do so for differing spiritual experiences. In these cases, they wish to achieve a deeper connection with the universe, enlightenment, have a greater understanding of the view they have on the world around them, and experience a sense of ultimate joy, peace, and serenity.

Psychedelic Integration

Psychedelic experiences can often cause individuals to go through drastic life changes. Typically through an experience, one becomes more aware of themselves, their actions, and their surroundings, and light is brought to areas in their life they should or need to change. Some individuals can easily decipher the meaning behind what occurs through their psychedelic experience but many others, especially those who have never had an experience before, may find it more challenging to incorporate their experiences into their daily lives. Where do individuals go to help sort through their psychedelic experience and utilize what they learned from the experience into their daily lives? This is where psychedelic integration can be of great help.

Psychedelic integration refers to a coach, therapist, or counselor that assists individuals in understanding their psychedelic experiences. Psychedelic integration therapy can especially help individuals who have gone through a bad psychedelic experience. Through this type of therapy, individuals can gain insight into the feelings that have arisen since having a psychedelic experience.

Many individuals have positive experiences but may not fully understand how to utilize what they learned through the experience to guide them in a new direction in life. Psychedelic integration is a new method that has been gaining much attention from those who have had psychedelic experiences. There are already a number of psychedelic integration locations in the United States though not many make themselves known publicly. With new psychedelic drug approvals, more of these psychedelic integration sites are becoming public.

Psychedelic integration is a short-term process that works with individuals to discuss one experience at a time and focuses on harnessing growth. Client and therapist or coach will build trust so the client is able to feel more comfortable discussing their experience. Often this can be a long process for those who have had a bad experience as they may not be eager to open up and remember the experience again. Psychedelic integration sessions can sometimes use different techniques and methods to help clients feel more relaxed and peaceful, which can often help people feel more confident about sharing and become more open to understanding their experiences. Mindfulness, guided personal awakening, and combined intuition are some of these techniques.

What psychedelics integration also aims to do is to provide a new way for others to open up and embrace the possibilities of insight that can be gained from a psychedelic experience. They supply a resource to individuals that will allow them to gain more knowledge and information regarding psychedelics in general and their benefits. They cover precautions, safety tips, and provide tools to those who are considering having their own psychedelic experience that will allow them to reduce risk and harm during their experience. While technically it is still illegal to use psychedelics for personal growth reasons, many integration coaches are hesitant to supply clients with exactly how to go about having a psychedelic experience. Other integration coaches look at providing the information as a way to better ensure their client's safety.

If you are considering having your own psychedelic experience then going to psychedelic integration coach can be valuable. They can help answer questions individuals may have about the experience and help you prepare for the experience. It is a safe, judgment-free space that aims to help individuals make the best decisions for them as to whether or not a psychedelic experience can be beneficial.

Psychedelic Support Groups

Psychedelic support groups are designed to help individuals understand and find meaning from their psychedelic experience. These groups are often guided by psychedelic integration coaches, therapists, or counselors. These group settings are a further way to allow individuals to better understand the psychedelic experience in a supportive way. Psychedelic support groups provide individuals many of the same services that a psychedelic integration coach will provide except this is offered in a group setting.

In group meetings, individuals can share their psychedelic experience to gain feedback on how to translate the lesson learned into their daily lives. Psychedelic support groups are also a way to gain knowledge and understanding of psychedelics even more. It can be beneficial for those who are considering having their own psychedelic experience to attend a psychedelic support group to gain a better understanding of what to expect. By hearing the stories of others who have had experiences one can better prepare for their own experience. The psychedelic support group also ensures participants are aware of harm reduction techniques.

Many of these psychedelic support groups also discuss topics that include ways to better gain support for decriminalization and legalization of psychedelic drugs. Participants learn ways that they can educate others and spread honest awareness of the use and safety of psychedelic use. Often these psychedelic support groups will meet on a monthly or bi-monthly basis.

Chapter 14:

The Future of Psychedelic Use

There is a deep need and desire for more effective ways to treat a number of illnesses, especially those involving mental health. This is what is ultimately causing researchers and lawmakers to reconsider the ban on psychedelic drug testing and research. Though many studies and clinical trials have shown the highly effective results of using psychedelic drugs there are still years of trials that will need to be conducted before any are approved for use in the United States.

Future research

With organizations like MAPS and the Beckley Foundation, much progress is being made in research and testing of psychedelic drug treatment. These organizations help researchers obtain approval to do vital testing and clinical trials that will eventually lead to government officials and the public to be more aware and understand the benefits these drugs can have in the medical field. It is because of these foundations that MDMA has been pushed through various phases of clinical trials and testing. This has made it more likely that in the near future it will start to be utilized as an effective form of treatment to those suffering from various mental health disorders, especially those with PTSD. These organizations rely on private funding and support to pay for testing and clinical trials and have been a vital component to psychedelic drugs being viewed in a new positive light.

Aside from clinical trials and research being conducted, the Berkley and MAPS organizations host a number of events to not only educate people on psychedelic drugs but also to show scientific findings and new developments in the medical field in regard to the effective use of psychedelic drugs. With the help of these two groups and others, the future looks hopeful for many who could benefit from psychedelic drug treatment.

Many researchers are focusing on the way they can create drugs that will not have the same mind-altering effects as those caused by psychedelics. If they can create drugs that help increase the level of neurotransmitters, regrow neurons, and create more awareness, these types of drugs may be easier to obtain permission to test on. But, would removing the hallucinogenic qualities of the psychedelic make it as effective? One of the reasons these types of drugs have been shown to be effective is not just because of the way it changes the brain's physical structure, it is more so because of the way it can put patients at ease.

In therapy sessions that have utilized psychedelic drugs, one of the reasons patients saw such success is because they were finally able to confront, understand, and work through the repressed memories, thoughts and feelings they either did not know were there or struggled to accept before. Creating a drug that simply repairs the chemistry of the brain will only provide half the benefits that psychedelics provide to patients.

Psychedelic Therapists

There has been recent training available that allows one to become a specialized psychedelic therapist. In the United States, becoming a psychedelic therapist can prepare you for the possibility of MDMA being made a legal form of medical treatment by 2021. Psychedelic therapists will soon be in great demand. Previously it was possible to become a trained psychedelic therapist, but in the United States, you could not practice if you were involved in a clinical trial that tested psychedelic drugs. Since the most successful trial is in its last phase it won't be long before many psychedelic clinics will be sought out.

Some states already offer training in psychedelic-assisted training, like at the California Institute of Integral Studies.

In order to be granted permission into the program, you must already be a licensed medical professional. The training is believed to cover classic psychedelics as well as newer psychedelic drugs. Much time is spent on furthering the understanding of the states of consciousness, the history of psychedelics, and philosophical areas. They also combine residential training with in-person and online coursework. The training tends to go on for about nine months and also provides participants with guest lectures and participation in week-long retreats.

MAPS also offers specific training on becoming an MDMA psychedelic therapist. Through their training, they require participants to pair up with another person who is licensed to practice psychotherapy. Each individual is expected to be trained in therapeutic therapy, ethics, trauma, and relationship therapy, though one person in the pair does not have to be actually licensed. They also require a prescribing physician who is able or has already obtained a license for MDMA be employed at their clinic. Training through MAPS focuses specifically on MDMA as opposed to the various psychedelic drugs like the California Institute of Integral Studies, and being approved for the training program can be incredibly difficult. Individuals wishing to take part in the training must meet a list of qualifications. Once accepted, participants are allowed one dose of MDMA to test on themselves but must give data and feedback to be included as research for the clinical trial being run at the time. Participants are not required to take a dose of MDMA but it can be beneficial as a way to better understand the drug and its effects. The participants are responsible for administering in their own clinics once MDMA is approved by the FDA.

Media Portrayal

The reason psychedelic drugs so easily and quickly gained a bad reputation is because of the various negative images and portrayals of those who use psychedelic drugs shown in the media. Media and advertisement allowed anti-drug and negative connotations of psychedelic drugs to spread to the masses within minutes. It was able to instantly create panic among the population which resulted in immediate demand that drastic measures be taken to protect the safety of the people.

Often times these early depictions of psychedelic use were associated as being the same as that of heroin or cocaine. The "this is your brain on drugs" commercial could be heard on every television set. What wasn't being talked about was how the drugs they pointed the finger at for causing the younger generation to rebel, were the drugs that could have helped treat the numerous addictions caused from already prescribed drugs. Those drugs they thought would fry their brains were actually the ones that could help regrow neurons and improve brain function. The drugs that caused such a divide in a country that was already divided and plagued with corruption and defeat, were the drugs that could have allowed for more peace, understanding, and compassion. No one was talking about the breakthroughs that were being made with these drugs, they were just focusing on the negative views and experience of the few and not the majority.

Today, media can have the same impact, but in a positive manner when it comes to talking about psychedelic drugs. The more psychedelic testing and results being shared and the more the misconceptions being addressed and corrected, the more the public opinion and views of these drugs will change. Because it is much easier for individuals to gain knowledge and learn about psychedelic use it won't be long before more of the population see the benefits of psychedelic drug treatment.

Not only is the media, in general, looking at psychedelics in a less negative manner, but it is also apparent in many news broadcasts and articles you can find. Whereas in the past, news stations and articles tended to have an underlying tone of not supporting psychedelic use, more of them now approach the topic in a matter-of-fact way.

Changes in the Law

When cannabis, or CBD, was made available for medicinal purposes this opened the doors for researchers to push to get permission to further test other psychedelic drugs for medicinal use. Ketamine is now being used to help treat depression, CBD is also being used to treat epilepsy, so what's next? How can more of these drugs make their way into the medical field? What would make it easier for more testing to be conducted is addressing the classification system that is in desperate need of updating? What can also continue to be done is what was done when cannabis first started to be decriminalized, is that states can take it into their own hands to change the laws around psychedelic drugs.

States like California and Denver are leading the way in this movement. In 2019, Denver voters went to the polls to decide whether or not psilocybin should be legal in the state, the result of this vote decriminalized psilocybin as well as other psychoactive plants. California plans to come out with a ballot that will also decriminalize psilocybin and allow for it to be used for both medical and religious purposes. Vermont and Oregon have also taken steps to allow psilocybin sessions to be conducted under professional supervision.

These are great advancements that have occurred in just a few years. Considering how in 2016 most of the United States population still strongly opposed any form of psychedelic legalization, this gives great hope that change will come swiftly.

With MDMA likely to be the next psychedelic to be approved for medicinal use by 2021 it is very likely that many more states will be moving forward with decriminalizing different psychedelics.

What one must keep in mind, as new advancements regarding psychedelic drug use is made, we cannot and should not compare the present moment to that of the 60s when psychedelics were used frequently for recreational purposes. In the 60s, psychedelics were used in opposition to societal norms. "Hippies" did not promote the use of LSD, cannabis, or psilocybin just to get high, they did so because they knew the experience would bring about more awareness in individuals and could ultimately unify the population. These views of the world were greatly misunderstood. Mindfulness, meditation, universal laws? Talk like this was considered nonsense and even insane. Today, these ideas are greatly accepted in society. Mediation, yoga, spiritual retreats, are all encouraged as a way to live a more fulfilled life. Psychedelics are the same. Most of the negative perception that surrounds psychedelics was initially from a lack of understanding or resistance to embracing a new way of understanding the world. Much of the resistance for legalizing psychedelic use comes from the fear of seeing the world being overrun as it apparently was in the 60s. But there are additional factors to take into consideration and one cannot ignore that what so many young adults were rebelling against in the 60s are of no concern today.

With new discoveries and testing being done it seems as though psychedelic drugs can open a doorway to more effective treatment. With an understanding of how psychedelic compounds directly affect neuron structure and cell growth, scientists can begin to work on a way to extract the compounds that have a direct effect on brain function while excluding the components that cause hallucinations and sensory distortions. However, more research is necessary to understand the extent of this effect and the limitations that would have to be imposed.

What research needs to focus on

While psychedelic drugs give adults a more hopeful outlook for treating mental illnesses and disorders, the same outlook might not be possible for children or young adults suffering from these conditions as well. Since children's brains are still developing, it is unclear how prompting cellular growth in their growing brains can affect them in the long-term. It is already known that those on the spectrum of being at a greater risk of suffering from a mood or psychological disorder, already have an increase in the number of mTORs activated in their brain.

Research also needs to focus more on the long-term effects of psychedelics. While this form of treatment will not require as frequent or even high doses of psychedelic drugs, understanding and knowing what, if any, long-term effects can be expected can possibly help gain more support in research efforts and FDA approval.

It is questionable whether it is necessary to research the benefits that younger children may gain from psychedelics. While they are safe for most adults, many children are still going through a number of changes. If anything, more research would need to be focused on how increased neural growth and increased levels of neurotransmitters can have an impact on developing brains. Additionally, being unable to control exactly what type of experience an individual has should also be considered in regard to children and psychedelics. If an adult has a bad experience they can simply come of the high, accept that it was just the drugs, and go about their daily lives. If a child has a bad experience this may lead to a greater risk of mental disorders and behavioral issues.

Final Considerations

What needs to be addressed is the common concern of the long-term effect of continued use of psychedelic drugs. Here is where there is another great misunderstanding. Individuals are typically used to having to take medications for various illnesses, conditions, disorders, and diseases for a prolonged period of time, even for the rest of their life. All these drugs being prescribed today have negative effects, many more serious than those short term negative effects of psychedelic drugs, and even the long-term effects that are known are not as severe as some of those of prescription drugs. Most patients who are on prescription drugs will eventually need to be prescribed another medication to help alleviate symptoms that the first prescribed drug causes.

Individuals who suffer from mental disorders often look at these prescriptions as chains. Those with chronic pain conditions look at their medication as cages, since many cause fatigue. Taking these medications may help alleviate symptoms but it also brings about other side effects that still hinder their ability to go about their day as they would like to. These medications do little to improve their quality of life. While some medications can be highly beneficial and effective, would an alternative that would allow individuals to stop having to take a pill every day be more appealing?

The main difference between using psychedelic drugs over traditional drugs is that in just about every study conducted, the positive effects and reduction of symptoms were immediately experienced and lasted for months after one low dose. There is no need to take psychedelic drugs every day or every week, and this point seems to be overlooked when weighing the pros and cons of how beneficial a drug can be. The first defense is that the long-term effects of continual psychedelic drug use cause other health problems, again, not unlike drugs already being prescribed. What this line of defense does not acknowledge is that many patients will only need to receive one dose, and many others may not need to receive another dose for years after the first. This is hardly continuous use of the drug and therefore the negative side effects of continuous use are not of much concern.

In this case, do the benefits of psychedelic drugs outweigh the possible negative effects? The answer is a matter of opinion, and it is hard to know just what the long-term effects are as psychedelic drug use is still fairly new. However, it would be hard to deny or admit that psychedelic drug treatment can be a much more affordable and effective form of treatment for many individuals who have suffered long enough.

Conclusion

Before they were banned, psychedelic drugs showed great promise in changing the way many mental health conditions could be treated. Because of a political agenda, all that promise and hope was lost. Luckily, a number of researchers still believed in the potential that psychedelic drugs could provide a viable and highly effective form of treatment.

If you look back in history you can find evidence of psychedelic drugs being used because of their healing properties as well as transcendental experiences. From the deserts in Mexico to the forest of the Amazon, psychedelics have been around long before LSD was engineered. These potent plants that were used in rituals and ceremonies shed light on not just the experience but the possibilities.

For decades, research around psychedelics slowed significantly, but a group of researchers in the 1990s and 2000s revisited the possibilities of psychedelic treatments. Through the support of various organizations like MAPS and the Beckley Foundation, hundreds of trials and vital research was conducted to show the benefits and effectiveness of psychedelic drugs.

Because of this persistence, a few of these drugs have finally been approved as a form of treatment. Though there is still a long way to go before many of these drugs will gain approval it at least gives hope that researchers are on the right path.

Much of the resistance that is revolved around psychedelics is because of public opinion on these types of drugs. This book has given you scientific evidence that shows how useful they can be in the medical field and for personal growth. Though no drug can ever be said to be 100% safe, as there are always going to be individuals who abuse drugs, this book reveals that safety concerns of psychedelic drug use are all misconceptions. Previously held opinions of psychedelic drugs are changing as more scientific evidence is being gathered, therefore, if you had a negative opinion of these drugs you now have a better understanding that these drugs are not like many of the others they tend to be compared with.

This book has covered a number of topics that have given you a starting point towards understanding psychedelics more. Maybe it has changed your opinion, maybe it has sparked more interest, or maybe it has clarified things more. Hopefully, you have gained a new perspective and a more open mind on the subject of psychedelics and it is one that you will share to help spread a better understanding of these valuable drugs.

www.ingramcontent.com/pod-product-compliance
Lightning Source LLC
Chambersburg PA
CBHW051345280526
45784CB00007B/2822